Anti-Inflammation Diet

FOR

DUMMIES®

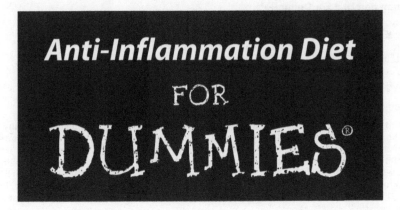

Anti-Inflammation Diet

FOR

DUMMIES®

by Artemis Morris, ND, LAc and Molly Rossiter

WILEY

John Wiley & Sons, Inc.

Anti-Inflammation Diet For Dummies®

Published by
John Wiley & Sons, Inc.
111 River St.
Hoboken, NJ 07030-5774
www.wiley.com

WILEY

About the Authors

Dr. Artemis Morris is a naturopathic physician, licensed acupuncturist, teacher, researcher, writer, and consultant on nutrition and holistic medicine. She completed her naturopathic doctorate and master's in acupuncture at Bastyr University in Seattle, Washington and has been in practice for over 10 years. Artemis is the medical director and founder of Revive Wellness Center, an integrative medicine practice in New Haven, Connecticut, and she has a private practice in Milford, Connecticut. She has served as the medical director for the Integrative Wellness Center at Masonic Healthcare Center in Wallingford, Connecticut.

Artemis teaches clinical nutrition at the University of Bridgeport College of Naturopathic Medicine and teaches nutrition and traditional Chinese medicine for an integrative master's degree program in Connecticut.

Artemis specializes in clinical nutrition, herbal medicine, acupuncture, diabetes, and women's healthcare. She is devoted to education, research, and writing in natural medicine, nutrition, ethnobotany, and the safe and effective use of nutritional supplements.

Molly Rossiter is an award-winning writer with more than 20 years of experience in journalism, most recently as the Faith & Values reporter for *The Gazette* (Cedar Rapids, Iowa), one of the top 200 newspapers in the U.S. with an Audit Bureau of Circulations-certified readership between 150,000 and 200,000 daily. As part of her beat, she regularly covers new research and interviews experts in various fields including science and religion and methods to improve one's sense of well-being.

Her journalism honors include awards from the Iowa Associated Press Managing Editors, the Association for Women in Communications, and the Iowa Newspaper Association. She was on the *Gazette* staff as it was being considered for a Pulitzer Prize in community journalism for its work covering the devastating floods of 2008.

A native of Iowa, Molly has lived in various parts of the country and is now back in her home state, where she lives with her two teenage children and two dogs.

Dedications

From Artemis: I dedicate this book to my patients. Thank you for sharing your experiences with me and helping me to perfect the secrets of a practical and truly healthy way of eating.

From Molly: I dedicate this book to my incredible teenagers, Justin and Kimberly. Thank you both for being such amazing people and having the patience and understanding that allowed me to work on this project.

Authors' Acknowledgments

From Artemis: Thank you to the team I have worked with on this book, the teachers I have had along the way, my patients, family, and students — it is through your interaction and collaboration that knowledge has turned to the wisdom contained in these pages. I hope that this book is a resource that inspires many to live a healthy and fulfilling life.

From Molly: Thank you to the incredible team I was able to work with on this book, and thanks to the many teachers and mentors I have had along the way. A special thanks to Meg and Barb, without whom this road would remain untraveled. I've learned many valuable lessons with this book and hope the words on these pages provide insight and healthier habits to those who read them.

Publisher's Acknowledgments

We're proud of this book; please send us your comments at http://dummies.custhelp.com. For other comments, please contact our Customer Care Department within the U.S. at 877-762-2974, outside the U.S. at 317-572-3993, or fax 317-572-4002.

Some of the people who helped bring this book to market include the following:

Acquisitions, Editorial, and Media Development

Project Editor: Elizabeth Rea

Acquisitions Editor: Michael Lewis

Senior Copy Editor: Danielle Voirol

Assistant Editor: David Lutton

Editorial Program Coordinator: Joe Niesen

Technical Editor: Deborah Lightstone, BSc, ND

Nutritional Analyst: Patricia Santelli

Recipe Tester: Emily Nolan

Editorial Manager: Michelle Hacker

Editorial Assistant: Alexa Koschier

Art Coordinator: Alicia B. South

Cover Photos: © iStockphoto.com/brebca

Cartoons: Rich Tennant (www.the5thwave.com)

Composition Services

Project Coordinator: Nikki Gee

Layout and Graphics: Samantha K. Cherolis, Nikki Gately, Corrie Socolovitch

Proofreader: Penny L. Stuart

Indexer: Christine Karpeles

Illustrators: Kathryn Born, Elizabeth Kurtzman

Special Help
Megan Knoll

Publishing and Editorial for Consumer Dummies

Kathleen Nebenhaus, Vice President and Executive Publisher

Kristin Ferguson-Wagstaffe, Product Development Director

Ensley Eikenburg, Associate Publisher, Travel

Kelly Regan, Editorial Director, Travel

Publishing for Technology Dummies

Andy Cummings, Vice President and Publisher

Composition Services

Debbie Stailey, Director of Composition Services

Contents at a Glance

Recipes at a Glance

Table of Contents

Introduction

‧ ‧

*T*here seems to be a diet for everything these days: one for improving heart health, one for detoxifying the body, one for bulking up, hundreds for slimming down. What if there were a diet designed to just make you feel better, relieve painful chronic illnesses, and even prevent the onset of future disease? The anti-inflammation diet is designed to do just that.

For years researchers have studied the impact certain foods have on people's digestive systems, but did you know they've also been watching the impact foods have on the muscles, bones, liver, kidneys, and other organs? What's more, physicians and researchers have discovered links between certain foods and chronic illnesses such as diabetes, cancer, rheumatoid arthritis, multiple sclerosis, and more — links that may be broken with an anti-inflammatory diet. Certain foods and food groups help promote inflammation in your body, just as others — such as fish, nuts, seeds, and organic fruits and vegetables — can help you avoid such diseases.

Anti-Inflammation Diet For Dummies serves as an introduction to the foods you should avoid and those that you should pile up, and it explains how you can change your lifestyle into one that's inflammation-free.

About This Book

This book is for anyone who is suffering from one of a multitude of chronic illnesses, for those who know someone who is suffering, and for people who simply want to avoid pain and discomfort in the future.

Diet plays a key role in how you feel, well beyond the fullness you feel after a big meal. Certain foods — refined sugars, foods high in saturated fats, and some meats — can actually work against your body and contribute to diabetes, heart disease, and cancer.

This book is a starter guide, an introduction to signs and symptoms of a variety of chronic illnesses and conditions related to inflammation. We introduce you to the healthiest foods, herbs, and supplements, and we steer you away from foods that can — and do — cause problems. We don't simply say, "This is bad"; we tell you why something is bad, why it's good, how it can help, or how it can further damage your tissues and cells.

We also help you put the anti-inflammation diet into practice. Not only does this book give you a list of the foods that are good, but it also features more than 100 easy-to-moderate recipes for almost any occasion, all geared toward stopping inflammation in its tracks. In addition, this book offers simple exercises and yoga positions to help you further move inflammation out of your life.

This book is a reference book, so you don't have to read everything or read everything in order. We designed it so you can jump in and read about whichever topics most interest you — or the ones that can offer you the most relief.

Conventions Used in This Book

Following are some conventions we use. Keep them in mind when reading this book:

- We discuss chronic illness and disease in basic and general terms. This book is not meant to be used in making any kind of diagnosis or to be a substitute for a visit to your physician or nutritional expert. Also, the foods we list in this book are a good start, but you should consult your naturopath or physician for a more complete list.

- Most of the recipes in Part III are not only anti-inflammatory but also designed for people suffering from lactose intolerance or gluten sensitivity. In recipes not designed for those people, we suggest substitutions you can make.

- In the recipes, all eggs are large, organic, and free-range. All the fresh fruits, vegetables, and herbs are organic as well to avoid pesticides and genetically modified ingredients. We offer the purest recipes with as little chemical interference as possible.

- The exercises and yoga positions listed in this book are good starter exercises for people who are just getting started. If you already subscribe to a workout regimen, step up the moves or push yourself just a little harder by taking a class, trying a tougher workout, or simply extending the time of your own workout.

- We use *italics* for terms that we define and **bold** for keywords or phrases in bulleted lists. Web addresses appear in `monofont`.

What You're Not to Read

Sidebars (text enclosed in shaded gray boxes) give you information that enhances but is not vital to the chapters in which they appear. You can skip them if you're pressed for time and not worry about missing out on the most important information. You can also skip any text marked by a Technical Stuff icon. That info is interesting but not essential to your understanding.

Foolish Assumptions

In writing this book, we made some assumptions about you, the reader:

- You aren't a medical doctor, so you don't need highly technical information. You're using this book as a guide to better, healthier living.

- You or someone close to you suffers from inflammation and you're interested in knowing ways to curb the pain and discomfort without the need for an arsenal of medication. Or you don't want to suffer from arthritis, diabetes, multiple sclerosis, or cancer later on in life and are looking for something to keep chronic disease at bay.

- You're interested in changing your diet, whether it's a complete overhaul or just substituting some healthier options for some of the not-so-healthy foods in your diet now.

How This Book Is Organized

This book contains six parts, consisting of 22 chapters and two appendixes. Throughout the book, we include cross-references to other parts of the book to make it easy for you to get a fuller understanding of a certain subject, but each part and chapter stands on its own, so you can read in any order that you like.

Part I: Taking the Mystery Out of Inflammation

In this part, we offer the basic definition of inflammation and discuss both the good side and the bad side of inflammation. We point out the various ways inflammation first works to defend the body against invaders — viruses, bacteria, and injuries that trigger the immune system.

This part also introduces the relationship between food and chronic illness. We define toxic foods and note how these foods can create problems in your body. We identify some of the chronic illnesses affected by or caused by inflammation and offer guidance on which foods may help you manage the symptoms.

Part II: Understanding Anti-Inflammatory Nutrition

Here's where we get down to the nitty-gritty. Not only do we break foods down categorically — which foods fare better on the anti-inflammation food pyramid, for example — but we also note how each food activates the vitamins and nutrients in others. We talk about different kinds of proteins and fats, noting which ones you need and which ones you need to avoid. We also take a look at carbohydrates and all the buzz around them: Are they good, are they bad, do they matter? (*Hint:* The answer is yes, yes, and yes.)

Part III: Enjoying Recipes for Less Inflammation and Better Health

This part is the fun part of the book, where we offer recipes ranging from breakfast bowls to dessert dishes, all with a goal of keeping inflammation away. The best part about these recipes is that virtually anyone with any kind of experience in the kitchen can put them together — you don't need to be the next top chef or have a commercial kitchen to make healthy fare.

Though not everyone looking for an anti-inflammation diet has sensitivities or allergies to dairy or wheat, many of these recipes are dairy- and gluten-free, or we note ways to make them so.

Part IV: Living an Anti-Inflammatory Lifestyle

Here's where we really get you ready to stick to your anti-inflammation diet. In this part, we discuss what needs to come out of your pantry and fridge and which types of foods, herbs, spices, and beverages you should restock them with. We then highlight different ways to cook food, because cooking a good food the wrong way can make it inflammatory. Here we show you how to — and how not to — prepare your foods.

Of course, switching to an anti-inflammation diet doesn't mean you're chained to your kitchen. In this part, we also talk about making wise choices when eating out, whether you're going to a nice sit-down restaurant or making the occasional stop at a fast-food place.

We also take a look at the various over-the-counter drugs and supplements designed to help deter inflammation. And we discuss exercises and yoga moves to help keep your heart and body healthy, because as with any kind of diet, exercise should be a key addition.

Part V: The Part of Tens

Want lists? We got 'em here, right at your fingertips. In this part, we give you ten benefits of stopping inflammation, ten inflammation-fighting foods, and ten anti-inflammation supplements and herbs, all with details indicating just why each item made the list.

Part VI: Appendixes

This part contains two appendixes to supplement your experience with the anti-inflammation diet. First is an explanation of the inflammation factor rating system and the inflammation index, two tools that help you determine the inflammatory properties of certain foods. We also provide a metric conversion chart for cooks who use the metric system.

Icons Used in This Book

Icons are the fancy little pictures in the margins of this book. Here's a guide to what they signify:

This icon gives you hints and suggestions, usually to make a good thing even better.

Here we draw your attention to key ideas you should remember even after you close the book.

Whenever you change your diet or start looking at medications and supplements, you should consult your doctor for precautions. This icon serves as a reminder in cases where you should exercise extra caution and/or get a medical opinion.

You see this icon attached to information that, although interesting, isn't vital to your understanding of the topic.

Where to Go from Here

You can start at the beginning and read straight through, or you can skip right to the recipes and find out why they're good for you later. Want to see how your dietary supplement compares to others? Skip straight to Chapter 22. Need some good exercises to go along with your healthy habits? See Chapter 18. Trying to figure out how many servings of something you should eat on a daily or weekly basis? Check out Chapter 4.

The great thing about this book is that order doesn't matter. If you need information in one chapter to better understand another, you can jump back and forth, and we include cross-references where appropriate to help you get the whole picture, no matter where you start.

Part I

Taking the Mystery Out of Inflammation

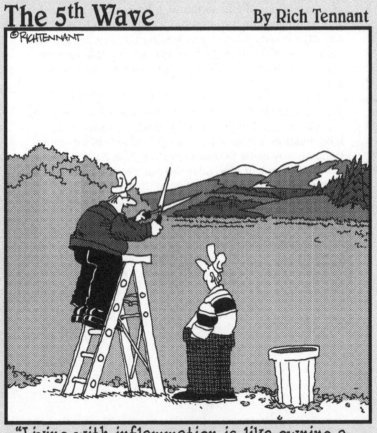

The 5th Wave   By Rich Tennant

"Living with inflammation is like owning a large hedge. The more you manage it, the better the outlook."

In this part . . .

In this part, we do just what the title says: We take the mystery out of inflammation. Inflammation is actually a good thing when it does what it's supposed to do, like seal off an injured area by providing swelling around the injury. But when the signals between your cells go haywire, inflammation becomes more of a hindrance than a help.

The chapters in this part take you inside inflammation to discover where it comes from and what causes good inflammation. We also discuss the bad side of inflammation and why some people seem to get hit harder than others. We look at food allergies and sensitivities, and we uncover the relationship between them and various chronic illnesses, such as cancer, diabetes, multiple sclerosis, and arthritis.

Chapter 1

Inflammation, Food, and You

* *

In This Chapter

▶ Understanding how inflammation fits into the immune system

▶ Using nutrition to decrease inflammation

▶ Making lifestyle changes beyond the food you eat

* *

*I*f you ever fell off your bike or out of a tree, you're familiar with inflammation surrounding an injury. In most cases, inflammation surrounds minor
cuts and bruises in the form of swelling and protects the injured area until it
heals. Since the late 1980s, however, researchers have turned their attention
to other causes of inflammation, such as diet and internal imbalances. These
inflammatory responses may be so severe that they lead to chronic illness,
such as diabetes, arthritis, heart disease, and cancer.

In this chapter, you get a better idea of just what inflammation is — both
the good and the bad — as well as how it's defined and what to look for.
Throughout the remainder of this book, you discover foods that may contribute to the problem as well as those foods, vitamins, and supplements that
may lessen the effects of inflammation.

What Is Inflammation?

The first thing you need to know about inflammation is that it's not all
bad. In fact, inflammation plays an important role in keeping you healthy.
Inflammation is the body's way of protecting itself from harmful bacteria,
viruses, and injury. In some cases, though, that system causes the body to
turn on itself, attacking healthy cells and organs. In this section, we take a
look at the various kinds of inflammation and identify how things can go
wrong.

Understanding how the immune system responds

The *immune system* is a complicated association of organs, tissues, and cells that work together to protect the body. Inflammation is part of your body's response when it feels it's in danger of infection or further injury.

There are three kinds of immunity:

- **Passive:** *Passive immunity* is a temporary immunity that comes from another body, such as from the mother through the placenta or breast milk. Passive immunity typically disappears 6 to 12 months after birth.

- **Innate:** *Innate immunity* is the immunity you were born with. Innate immunity includes barriers that keep invaders from entering your body, as well as inflammatory responses — coughing; producing tears, sweat, mucus, and additional stomach acid; swelling; and so on.

- **Acquired:** *Acquired immunity* develops in the presence of certain antigens. It develops as your body builds defenses against specific invaders, such as viruses that cause chicken pox and the common cold.

In this section, we cover innate and acquired immunity, the two immune systems that stick around through adulthood. We discuss inflammation as part of the innate immune system, and we cover the invader-specific defenses of the acquired immune system.

Innate immunity: Providing general protection with inflammation

Inflammation is part of your body's innate response to invaders. The inflammatory response takes over when harmful bacteria, viruses, toxins, or other elements make their way into your tissues and cause damage. Those damaged cells release chemicals called prostaglandins and histamines, which cause blood vessels to leak fluid into the tissues and create swelling.

The resulting inflammation — characterized by redness, swelling, heat, and pain — serves as a physical barrier against the spread of infection (in the case of illness) or against further injury (which would delay the healing process). Chemical factors released during inflammation ward off or sensitize pain signals, creating a more suitable environment for healing.

Meanwhile, the immune system, sensing danger, sends backup. Various parts of the immune system respond by directing traffic, isolating and killing the invaders, and destroying and clearing out infected cells. The cells communicate with each other through a variety of chemical signals, including cytokines, C-reactive protein, acute-phase proteins, prostaglandins, and

more. Understanding this response is helpful for doctors because inflammatory markers indicate where the problem is and how severe it may be.
Researchers examine the process to determine what triggers inflammation
and find ways to control it — such as through diet — when things go wrong.

Acquired immunity: Attacking specific invaders from past encounters

The acquired, or adaptive, immune system is the one you develop based on
what you do, where you go, and what you're exposed to. The more bugs and
viruses you come in contact with, the more complex your acquired immune
system becomes.

Through a process called *immune response,* the immune system calls upon
its network — cells, tissues, and organs — to combat illness and infection.
Leukocytes, or white blood cells, seek out and destroy infectious organisms
and substances. There are two kinds of leukocytes:

- ✔ *Phagocytes,* which are the hungry leukocytes that eat the invaders
- ✔ *Lymphocytes,* which help the body identify and recognize attackers so it
  knows what to watch for later

Here's what happens: When your body detects antigens (the foreign substances), a group of cells get together and form a type of cell army to attack
the invader. Some of these cells produce *antibodies* that can lock onto the
specific antigens. The antibodies serve as tags, identifying the invader as an
enemy and targeting it for destruction.

Some of the antibodies continue to live in your body so they can immediately
attack if the same antigen is detected. The next time the antibodies encoun-
ter that antigen, they lock on and initiate an inflammatory response.

Seeing where inflammation goes wrong

When inflammation works right, it attacks the irritant — the virus, harmful
bacteria, or damaged cells. Sometimes, however, the body kicks into overdrive and launches an offensive on normal, healthy tissue. For example, if you
have the autoimmune disorder rheumatoid arthritis, you see some redness
and some swelling in the joints, with joint pain and stiffness. This reaction is
a sign that your body is trying to attack your joint tissue, which your body
mistakenly perceives as unfriendly.

Say your house is being overtaken by mosquitoes. You get some mosquito
spray, light a citronella candle, and keep a rolled-up newspaper handy.
You're handling the irritant and the irritant only. Now say you've gone a little

bit overboard. Instead of a rolled-up newspaper, you take a baseball bat and try to kill that mosquito on the wall. The problem is that the mosquito wasn't a mosquito at all; it was just a shadow, and now you have a hole in the wall. In the same way, the immune system can overreact to perceived threats and damage the body.

The way your body responds to inflammation partially depends on your genetics and environmental factors. Most generally healthy people respond to a cut or bruise in the same way, but how the immune system responds to a virus, a bacteria, or different foods can differ from person to person. The differences in the way your immune system responds depends on the following:

- Your genes
- Your general state of health
- The health of major organs of immune function, such as the gastro-intestinal tract
- Dietary influences on health, including nutrients and toxins in food
- Environmental toxins, such as pesticides
- Blood sugar and insulin dysregulation
- Stress factors (stress weakens the immune system)

A major underlying factor in the different ways people are affected by inflammation is an imbalance in their acquired immune systems. In a healthy immune system, the *helper T cells* (those that are part of the immune response and attack) are in balance — one cell to attack blood-borne parasites, the other to attack invaders such as bacteria. As the immune system becomes overstimulated, the helper cells find themselves in a self-perpetuating imbalance, causing the helper cells to attack the body. As long as whatever is causing the inflammation is still present, the imbalance remains.

Inflammation can also go on too long. The innate and the acquired immune systems communicate with each other through sensors and signals, which tell the body when to release certain chemicals and proteins to activate the inflammation guard. The signals are supposed to tell the inflammation when to stop as well. That doesn't always happen. Some people have elevated levels of C-reactive protein, an inflammatory marker that leaves the body in defensive mode, always ready to attack. When that happens, your body begins a steady downward spiral leading to disease.

Creating inflammation isn't something your body does without effort — it takes energy, which causes fatigue and creates *free radicals,* molecules that cause cell damage. Thanks to all the things you're exposed to, cells related to the inflammatory response have to become pretty strong, which means that when they attack, they do so with force. That force can cause damage the longer those cells are active.

Understanding the difference between acute and chronic inflammation

Inflammation may be acute or chronic. The biggest difference between the two is time:

- ✔ **Acute:** *Acute inflammation* occurs almost immediately after tissue damage and lasts for a short time, from a few seconds to several days. It's what causes bruising and swelling when you fall or sprain something.

- ✔ **Chronic:** Although usually not as painful as acute inflammation, *chronic inflammation* lasts much longer, sometimes for several months. Chronic inflammation can be caused by physical factors (viruses, bacteria, blood sugar imbalances, extreme heat or cold) or emotional factors (chronic daily stress). Over time, chronic inflammation can contribute to chronic disease by throwing off the body's immune system and creating a lot more inflammation in the process.

Some researchers describe inflammation as *high-grade* or *low-grade,* depending on the severity of inflammation and the levels of inflammatory markers such as C-reactive protein (CRP). Low-grade inflammation, especially chronic low-grade inflammation, tends to be the more dangerous form. Low-grade inflammation often leads to chronic disease, such as atherosclerosis (hardened arteries), diabetes, cancer, arthritis, multiple sclerosis, irritable bowel syndrome, high blood pressure, and lupus. Many of the factors leading to low-grade inflammation are lifestyle-related: smoking, stress, obesity, inactivity, and diet.

Low-grade inflammation often goes undetected, but here are common symptoms:

- ✔ Body aches and pains
- ✔ Fever
- ✔ Congestion
- ✔ Frequent infections
- ✔ Stiffness
- ✔ Dry eyes
- ✔ Diarrhea or irritable bowel syndrome symptoms
- ✔ Indigestion
- ✔ Shortness of breath
- ✔ Fatigue

One of the first and best ways to determine whether you're experiencing low-grade inflammation is to have some blood work done. A healthcare professional can test your *highly sensitive-CRP* (hs-CRP) levels. According to the American Heart Association, an hs-CRP test can help determine a person's risk for heart disease, stroke, and other cardiac issues.

Gut reactions: Linking food, digestion, and the immune system

For you to remain healthy, your immune system must remain healthy and in balance. Getting the right kinds and amounts of proteins, fats, vitamins, and other nutrients is key in getting and staying healthy. Eating right gives your body the building blocks it needs to build cells and create chemicals, and the digestive system plays a key role in the immune system.

Breaking down food and dealing with the pieces

Digestion involves mechanical actions — the chewing and grinding of the food — as well as chemical processes, in which enzymes break down the food into tiny molecules. Your body puts these molecules through a selection process, keeping the useful molecules as raw materials for building cells, hormones, and so on; filtering out what it can't use; and neutralizing and removing harmful substances.

Eating the right kinds of foods in the right amounts ensures that your body has the raw materials it needs. For example, eating the right kinds of fats can strengthen your immune system and help you fight off inflammation. *Eicosanoids,* which are chemicals involved in inflammation, are made from essential fatty acids. Eating the right types of these fats, like omega-3 fatty acids, will allow your body to produce anti-inflammatory eicosanoids, something that doesn't happen when you eat too many omega-6 fatty acids. We discuss fats in Chapter 5.

Recognizing the digestive tract as part of the immune system

A major forgotten part of the immune system is the digestive tract. In fact, 80 percent of your immune system is found there. The digestive tract contains the *gut associated lymphoid tissue* (GALT), a type of tissue that monitors and protects the body against pathogens (germs). There is a high concentration of GALT in the small intestine, where your food gets absorbed.

Due to *oral tolerance,* the GALT doesn't respond to most foods you eat as foreign invaders. That's why you don't mount an immune system response to everything you eat. However, the GALT is the same part of the immune system that overreacts to food and mediates the hyperreactive immune response in food allergies, where the food is seen as an invader.

The intestines also offer a safe haven for beneficial bacteria, which aid in digestion and occupy prime real estate so other, harmful microorganisms can't move in. *Dysbiosis* is an imbalance of good and bad bacteria in the gut. Because many of its symptoms seem to be normal reactions to some foods, many people shrug off the condition. But if left untreated, it can turn into leaky gut syndrome, a major cause of disease.

Leaky gut syndrome is part of the mechanism that contributes to inflammation in the gastrointestinal (GI) tract and thus the rest of the body. Inflammation in the intestines disrupts the *tight junctions,* the glue that holds the cells of the intestines together in a self-contained tube. Most molecules are too big to fit through these junctions, so the only way for them to escape the intestines and enter the blood is to be ferried through the intestinal cells, from one side to the other. With inflammation, the junctions become "leaky" and let things such as large food particles and bacteria out into the rest of the body, where the immune system can attack them (see Figure 1-1). In this way, leaky gut syndrome, also known as *intestinal hyperpermeability,* contributes to autoimmune disorders, joint pains, and food allergies and sensitivities.

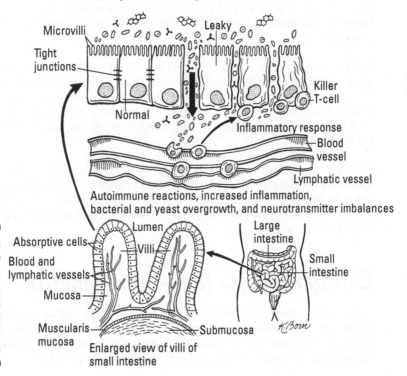

Infections, toxins, drugs and medications, stress, inflammatory diet, food allergies and sensitivities

Microvilli

Tight junctions

Leaky

Killer T-cell

Normal

Inflammatory response

Blood vessel

Lymphatic vessel

Autoimmune reactions, increased inflammation, bacterial and yeast overgrowth, and neurotransmitter imbalances

Lumen

Absorptive cells

Villi

Large intestine

Small intestine

Blood and lymphatic vessels

Mucosa

Muscularis mucosa

Submucosa

Enlarged view of villi of small intestine

Figure 1-1: With leaky gut syndrome, large particles can escape the digestive tract.

K. Born

Treating Your Symptoms with Nutrition

A lot of recent research has turned to the relationship between what people eat and how it affects their inflammation levels. Many foods common in most kitchens promote inflammation, and others have a noticeable diminishing effect on inflammation and may prevent it altogether.

In this section, we look at foods that can cause discomfort and how they're linked to inflammation. We tell you how to restructure your diet long-term to maintain good health and help you avoid sometimes-hidden internal inflammation.

Creating a diet that works for you

Creating an anti-inflammatory diet based on the foods your body accepts most helps you stay in good health while maintaining — or retaining — energy levels and ensuring you get an ample supply of vitamins and minerals.

Sometimes you may feel gassy or bloated or get a headache after eating, but have you ever stopped to think that it's a specific food that's causing those symptoms, and it very likely causes the same symptoms every time you eat it?

No one diet or menu works for everyone. Your needs are different from your neighbor's and different still from those of the person who lives down the street. If you're allergic to dairy products, it's a safe bet that foods made with cow's milk aren't going to top your list of foods to eat. People with celiac disease or gluten sensitivities aren't going to be eating a lot of breads or baked goods.

The first step in tailoring an anti-inflammatory diet is to determine which foods are good for *you* — which ones don't cause you pain, bloating, gas, or other feelings of discomfort. Read the list of toxic foods (see Chapter 2) to determine which foods to avoid and create a menu that helps your body and also tastes good.

Eating right for long-term benefits

Inflammatory foods can create instant symptoms as well as long-term effects. What's the damage in the long term? Inflammatory foods can speed the aging process, contribute to rheumatoid arthritis and other joint problems, and stimulate inflammation in a variety of ways (see Chapter 3).

Knowing which foods are inflammatory can be as simple as keeping one rule of thumb in mind: The less it looks like it did originally, the more inflammatory it likely is. Whole grains such as bulgur, brown rice, and oats all look like they do in the wild, complete with the germ and the entire grain kernel, so they're likely to be okay.

Whole, natural foods still contain many, if not all, of the vitamins and minerals they should have. Eating these foods is especially important for people with chronic diseases, genetic disorders, chronic stress, or metabolic disorders. These conditions increase the need for the vitamins and minerals that reduce inflammation and help the body work properly.

Splurging — or treating yourself — is okay now and then, but you should avoid certain inflammatory foods (see Chapter 4). Foods to avoid include high-omega-6 oils, such as those made from corn, safflower, sunflower, and cottonseed; inflammatory saturated fats from animal sources, as found in processed meats like bologna and hot dogs; trans fats; and refined sugars.

Striking the right nutritional balance is just as important as knowing which foods to eat. Make sure you're getting the right amount of proteins, healthy fats, vitamins and minerals, and other nutrients.

Supplementing Your Diet with an Anti-Inflammation Lifestyle

Creating an anti-inflammation diet is more than changing the foods you eat; it's committing to a change in lifestyle to give you a healthier life. Here are two areas of change that go hand-in-hand with the anti-inflammation diet:

- Restocking your kitchen with anti-inflammatory foods
- Relearning how to cook; if you're fond of deep-fried foods or even battered vegetables cooked in oil, get used to eating a little differently

Take a look at some of your habits or vices. Do you smoke? Drink? How much exercise do you get each day? Those are three big areas in which change — giving up smoking, reducing how much you drink, and increasing how much you exercise — can make a world of difference.

Physical activity helps with weight loss and maintenance, makes your heart work more efficiently, keeps your blood pressure in normal ranges, and reduces stress, a major factor in inflammation. Chronic stress depletes your body of the nutrients you need for your immune system to function properly. Get started with some meditation or yoga and take up a cardio workout to slow aging of the brain and build up your muscles and nerves. We discuss exercise and meditation in Chapter 19.

Chapter 2

Understanding How Food Can Be Your Body's Enemy

In This Chapter

▶ Identifying links between food and inflammation

▶ Knowing the difference between allergy and sensitivity

▶ Living with allergies and sensitivities

The first obstacle to get over when making a change to an anti-inflammatory diet is realizing that yes, some foods really *are* your enemy. Not all food is working against you, of course. But much of the food you consider safe, the foods that you may be eating regularly, may show up on your new do-not-eat list. After you identify your food allergies, sensitivities, and intolerances, keep them in mind as you select recipes and ingredients in later chapters.

Researchers have been working for years to determine how certain types of foods react with the human body and stir up inflammatory responses. It's no secret that fried foods, foods high in saturated fat, and those high in sugar are bad for you. What is surprising to many people, however, is the discovery that many of the foods that seem safe can really be hazardous to one's health, leading to sensitivities or allergies or even contributing to cancer, heart disease, or diabetes.

Defining Toxic Foods

Food, by definition, is "any nutritious substance that people eat or drink . . . in order to maintain life or growth." When you eat food, it becomes energy for your body through the process of digestion. The foods and drinks you take in aren't in a form that your bodies can use just yet; the food has to be transformed into much smaller pieces, nutrient-filled molecules, which can be absorbed by your blood and carried throughout the body. Digestion starts in the mouth as you chew food into smaller pieces; then it continues through the body with the help of digestive fluids until it's broken down as far as possible. Most of these molecules are absorbed into the small intestine and eventually become energy for various parts of the body.

Sometimes, however, that same food you turn to for nutrition and sustenance can turn on you. Foods that are seemingly harmless can be toxic, leading to inflammation and serving as triggers for chronic illnesses such as diabetes, cancer, arthritis, and heart disease.

We define *toxic foods* as any foods that are harmful to the body to any degree and can lead to inflammation and chronic disease. For some people, the *nightshade* family of fruits and vegetables — tomatoes, potatoes, peppers, eggplant — can be toxic in that they contain alkaloids, which can affect muscle function. Dairy products or wheat products can cause digestion problems for some people, and refined sugars can promote diabetes, obesity, and hypertension.

You can put toxic foods into three categories:

- ✔ Foods that increase inflammation in everyone, such as trans fats, refined sugars, and artificial foods

- ✔ Foods that are toxic to some individuals and not to others, such as wheat, corn, and dairy

- ✔ Foods that contain chemicals and other harmful substances that cause inflammation and endocrine changes in the body; they may accumulate in the fat cells and liver and can be associated with cancer

Toxic foods offer more harmful effects than healthy benefits. Refined sugar, trans fats, and bleached or enriched flour are the top three toxic foods for people seeking anti-aging strategies. Following is a sampling of some of the toxic foods found in everyday diets. We discuss these foods in detail in Chapter 4.

- ✔ **Refined sugars:**
  - Cookies, doughnuts, pastries
  - Prepared salad dressings and condiments
  - White bread
  - Pasta
  - Flavored oatmeal or cereal
  - Soda and fruit punch
  - Cereal bars

✔ **Trans fats:**

- French fries
- Margarine
- Packaged baked goods
- Potato and corn chips
- Fried foods
- Creamy salad dressings and condiments

✔ **Bleached or enriched flour:**

- Bread
- Crackers
- Cereal
- Cookies, even homemade
- Pasta
- Pancakes, waffles

Looking at Allergies and Specific Sensitivities

For many people, creating a menu isn't as simple as going with whatever they like to eat. People who have food allergies, sensitivities, or intolerances have to avoid foods and food products that many people take for granted.

✔ **Food allergies** are caused by an overreaction of the immune system toward a food or drink. Allergic reactions tend to show up almost immediately, from a rash or watery eyes to a more serious anaphylactic reaction that could be fatal.

✔ **Food sensitivities** appear in the form of a more delayed, sometimes chronic onset of symptoms, such as fatigue or even nasal congestion days after consumption. Food sensitivities are often caused by nutrient deficiencies or eating or drinking the food too often.

✔ **Food intolerance** is an adverse reaction to a food because something necessary for digestion is missing. For example, if your body is missing lactase, the enzyme needed to break down lactose, you're likely intolerant of milk and dairy products.

It can sometimes be difficult to distinguish between a hypersensitivity and an allergy to a food, as seen in Figure 2-1. Many of the same symptoms may appear with both hypersensitivity and allergies, but the chronic effects may differ. Consult a health care professional to determine if you have food allergies, sensitivities, or intolerances.

In this section, we take a look at various allergies, sensitivities, and intolerances; note some foods that commonly cause problems; and discuss how those food reactions can lead to chronic inflammation.

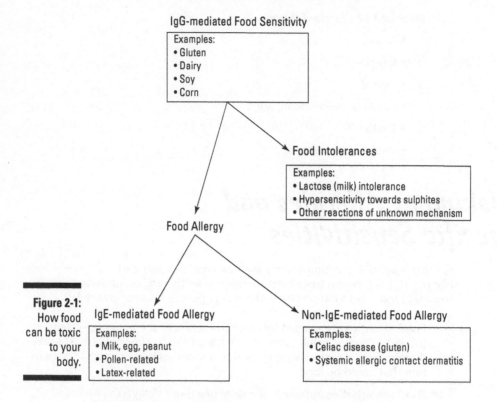

IgG-mediated Food Sensitivity

Examples:
• Gluten
• Dairy
• Soy
• Corn

Food Intolerances

Examples:
• Lactose (milk) intolerance
• Hypersensitivity towards sulphites
• Other reactions of unknown mechanism

Food Allergy

IgE-mediated Food Allergy

Examples:
• Milk, egg, peanut
• Pollen-related
• Latex-related

Non-IgE-mediated Food Allergy

Examples:
• Celiac disease (gluten)
• Systemic allergic contact dermatitis

Figure 2-1:
How food can be toxic to your body.

Understanding food allergies and sensitivities

Food allergies and sensitivities aren't all that uncommon. In fact, you may have an allergy and not even realize it. Allergies of all kinds occur when a body's immune system kicks in, attacking the irritant that it views as an invader.

Most of the time, your body doesn't attack the food you eat because of *food tolerance,* which is regulated by the immune system and your gastrointestinal tract. But as you age and practice more inflammatory habits, you can develop intolerances, sensitivities, or even life-threatening allergies to specific foods. Your immune system starts attacking either because too much of a particular component of that food is present or because there's something wrong with the way that food affects your body due to your genetic predisposition.

After the body first identifies — or rather, misidentifies — a particular food particle as an invader, the body starts mass-producing antibodies. When you eat something you're allergic to, antibodies lock onto an antigen (the offending food particle) and trigger an inflammatory response. In most cases, the inflammation quiets down again; however, if you have a genetic predisposition to food allergies, high levels of toxicity, digestive system imbalances, or a weakened immune system, this normal immune response can kick into high gear and wreak inflammatory havoc in your body in varying degrees.

Think of a bee sting. Everyone has some level of irritation or sensitivity to the stinger, even if it's not a full allergy. When the bee stings your arm, there's a small red bump where your antibodies immediately attack the area and work to protect the rest of the body. The same thing happens with food allergies and sensitivities, only the inflammation comes in the form of arthritis, irritable bowel syndrome, or other issues.

Food allergies and sensitivities can be lethal. Some people must avoid not only the product itself but also anything that may contain that product in its ingredients list. People allergic to peanuts, for example, have to avoid anything made with peanut oil. In extreme cases, people must even avoid foods that have come into contact with their allergen.

Addressing lactose intolerance

Most people have some degree of sensitivity to dairy, although the majority don't even realize it. About 30 percent of all Americans suffer from *lactose intolerance,* the inability to digest *lactose,* which is the main sugar found in milk. Some researchers go as far as saying that as much as 60 percent of the world's population can't digest milk and that being able to digest milk beyond infancy may be considered abnormal.

To be digested properly, the sugar lactose must be split into the smaller pieces glucose and galactose. When the *lactase* enzyme is either absent or inactive in the body, you can't break down lactose, and you have lactose intolerance. The body produces less lactase as you age, and in Asian, Native American, and African American populations, lactase production drops anywhere from 70 to 100 percent from childhood.

That's not to say everyone with a lactase deficiency is lactose intolerant; many people may go years without having any symptoms, or there may be just certain dairy products that trigger symptoms while others don't have any affect at all. But whenever you eat or drink something your body doesn't like, it sends out warning signals, usually in some form of inflammation. The most common symptoms of dairy sensitivity are gastrointestinal issues, but other symptoms with a potential relationship to dairy include

- ✔ Abnormal cravings for sweets
- ✔ Achy joints and muscles
- ✔ Acne
- ✔ Anxiety
- ✔ Bags under the eyes
- ✔ Chest congestion
- ✔ Chronic fatigue
- ✔ Dizziness or faintness
- ✔ Excessive sweating
- ✔ Headaches
- ✔ Mood swings
- ✔ Ulcers

Symptoms generally appear anywhere from 20 minutes to two hours after eating or drinking dairy products. Consume too much dairy, and symptoms can worsen, leading to abdominal distention and diarrhea as well as many other stomach problems.

If you suspect you may have lactose intolerance because you're experiencing any of the symptoms listed, look for the word *lactose* listed in the ingredients of some of your favorite foods — even those you may not think have any dairy. Be sure to get a proper diagnosis so you can rule out any other conditions that may be present.

People who have lactose intolerance can generally tolerate yogurt or other fermented dairy products because they contain helpful live organisms (*probiotics*) that help with digestion and healing the gastrointestinal system.

Confronting sugar and caffeine sensitivity

Refined sugar — which has been processed and stripped of all its natural nutrients — is bad for everyone. Unfortunately, that's also the type of sugar that's found in almost everything you eat. Refined sugar is much too easy to digest, so it quickly enters the bloodstream and raises blood sugar levels, increasing your risk of diabetes. Eat too much sugar, and you quickly see some symptoms of a suppressed immune system: fatigue, joint pain, confusion, forgetfulness. These symptoms can show up within just a day or two of eating a lot of sugar and yet may not be linked to sugar for years.

Sugar affects the body's insulin levels and can lead to insulin resistance over time, especially when you take in too much. With *insulin resistance,* the cells in the body have trouble responding to insulin and taking in glucose (blood sugar); when the glucose level in your bloodstream is elevated, it becomes much harder for your body to work. Obvious symptoms of sugar sensitivity are weight gain and pain in the joints.

Artificial sweeteners often aren't a good substitute for sugar. In many cases, you're simply replacing one bad thing with another. Instead of using processed sugar cane or sugar beets, you're consuming the chemicals and preservatives found in sweeteners. We discuss sugar, artificial sweeteners, and natural sweeteners in Chapter 8.

You know caffeine as the chemical you turn to when you need a quick pick-me-up or something to help you wake up in the morning. What you probably *don't* think about is the other effects that caffeine has on your body. At the same time caffeine is alerting your senses and awakening your mind, caffeine is creating a small rise in your blood sugar. That's not a big deal for a lot of people, but for people with diabetes, caffeine can turn a simple can of soda into a somewhat toxic cocktail. Caffeine becomes dangerous because it works to increase insulin resistance. (*Note:* Interestingly enough, although caffeine may have negative effects on the body's blood sugar levels, coffee and tea have both been shown to raise insulin sensitivity and lower blood sugar levels.)

Like the taste of that tea but want to lower the caffeine level? Dip the tea bag into hot water once, and then pour the water out. Refill the cup with hot water and continue dipping the teabag. The highest concentration of caffeine comes out with that first dip, so although you'll still have some caffeine, the level will be lower.

Watching wheat: Looking at celiac disease and gluten sensitivity

To many people, a piece of toast or a bagel for breakfast is a great way to start the day. For people with celiac disease and gluten sensitivity, it can be the start of a day filled with pain and discomfort. Everything made with wheat, barley, or rye is off-limits; even the smallest temptation can cause damage to the small intestine and related health problems.

Celiac disease and associated disorders

Celiac disease is an inherited autoimmune condition that affects both children and adults. It has to do with *gluten,* the protein found in all forms of wheat — including durum, semolina, spelt, khorasan (Kamut), einkorn, and faro — and related grains, such as rye, barley, and triticale. People with celiac disease have to avoid all foods that contain gluten.

When people with celiac disease eat gluten, it creates a reaction that damages the *villi,* the nutrient-absorbing projections on the lining of the small intestines. Because the body can't absorb the nutrients, someone with celiac disease may become malnourished. Even the smallest amount of gluten can pose a threat to people with celiac disease.

Celiac disease can develop at any time, from infancy to adulthood. Although damage to the villi may heal — it takes three to six months to heal in children, two to three years for adults — the person with celiac disease must continue to follow a gluten-free diet for the rest of his or her life.

Some of the symptoms of celiac disease are fatigue, bloating, constipation, weight loss, abdominal pain, gas, diarrhea, and weakness. It can progress to anemia, irritable bowel syndrome, and even early-onset osteoporosis.

Health problems that accompany celiac disease go well beyond the gastrointestinal tract. Damage to the bowels can lead to other *autoimmune disorders* (disorders that occur when the body's immune system attacks healthy tissue). Some associated autoimmune disorders, according to the Celiac Disease Foundation (CDF), are

- Insulin-dependent type 1 diabetes mellitus
- Liver diseases
- Thyroid disease — Hashimoto's thyroiditis
- Graves' disease
- Lupus (SLE)

- ✔ Addison's disease
- ✔ Chronic active hepatitis
- ✔ Rheumatoid arthritis
- ✔ Sjögren's syndrome
- ✔ Raynaud's syndrome
- ✔ Alopecia areata
- ✔ Scleroderma

In addition, several other disorders have been associated with celiac disease:

- ✔ Down syndrome
- ✔ Fibromyalgia
- ✔ Chronic fatigue syndrome
- ✔ Williams syndrome

Nonceliac problems with gluten

Some people have sensitivities to gluten and gluten products without having celiac disease. Nonceliac gluten sensitivity may occur when a person is eating a diet with excessive gluten and gluten products, increasing the risk that gluten protein fragments will get into the bloodstream.

Leaky gut syndrome, or increased permeability of the small intestines, is a defect in the barrier between the small intestines and the bloodstream. That defect allows harmful proteins to go directly into the bloodstream without being broken down as they should. The body then looks at those escaped proteins as foreign invaders.

The same autoimmune disorders that can be traced to celiac disease have links to leaky gut syndrome. Some more minor ailments caused by leaky gut syndrome include irritability, sluggishness, tiredness, achiness, and a decline in mental acuteness.

Avoiding gluten

Shopping for a gluten-free diet has become easier thanks to increased awareness of gluten sensitivities, but it's still a difficult task. Many grocery stores stock a gluten-free section, but that area is seldom more than a few shelves.

At the top of the list of foods to avoid are those made with wheat — which encompasses quite a lengthy list. Anything that contains flour generally contains wheat flour, even if it's not a whole-wheat item. Wheat can even be lurking in unexpected places — it's used as a thickening agent and is in a lot of condensed soups, gravy mixes, and sauces as well as in processed meats.

People who have gluten sensitivity or celiac disease also need to avoid foods and products made with barley and rye, which are relatives of wheat. Oats are naturally gluten-free, but they're often farmed on land on a rotation with wheat and are processed by the same machines, so look for a brand labeled "gluten-free" — Red Mill is a good brand. For more information on celiac disease and avoiding gluten, check out *Living Gluten-Free For Dummies* by Danna Korn (John Wiley & Sons, Inc.).

Getting Tested for Allergies and Sensitivities

Although everyone's allergy or sensitivity is different, some foods cause problems more often than others. Some of the most common food allergens are eggs, milk, soy and soy products, wheat, fish, shellfish, tree nuts, and peanuts. People with food allergies should also be cautious about eating other foods from the same evolutionary family. For example, people with wheat allergies need to be careful with other grains.

Some common food sensitivities are cow's milk, wheat and gluten, soy and soy products, peanuts, corn, eggs, chicken, pork, corned beef, oranges, strawberries, and tomatoes and other nightshade vegetables.

Figuring out what you're allergic or sensitive to, and what kind of reaction you have, is an important step in regaining and maintaining health and quality of life. When talking about food allergies and sensitivities, people are most often referring to either immunoglobulin E (IgE) or immunoglobulin G (IgG) allergies/sensitivities. The differences between the two lie in reaction time and severity:

- **IgE allergy:** An IgE allergy triggers the IgE antibody, which causes an immediate response when the offending substance enters the body. The people who are so severely allergic to peanuts that exposure even to peanut dust can be fatal have an IgE allergy, or *classic allergy*. Reactions include swelling, hives, difficulty breathing, and even anaphylactic shock.

- **IgG allergy/sensitivity:** With IgG allergies/sensitivities, the IgG antibody response is typically much more delayed and can include headaches, nausea, fatigue, and/or other digestive symptoms and even seizures. These allergies/sensitivities can also contribute to long-term health issues such as irritable bowel syndrome, diabetes, rheumatoid arthritis, and heart disease.

Three basic types of tests, done by a health care professional, can determine whether you have a food allergy:

- ✔ **Blood test:** The *radioallergosorbent test* (RAST) is a blood test that's generally conducted after a person has a recurring reaction to a particular food or foods. Signs of a possible allergic reaction to food are similar to other allergy signs: red or itchy eyes, hives, dermatitis (skin inflammation), coughing or sneezing, or stomach discomfort and diarrhea. A positive test doesn't determine how severe a reaction to a certain food may be, only that you may have a reaction of some kind.

- ✔ **Skin test:** A skin test, in which the skin is pricked, punctured, or scratched after coming in contact with a potential allergen, may show preliminary signs of allergy.

- ✔ **Food elimination test:** The elimination test is just as it sounds — a test for allergies conducted by first eliminating all possible allergens from your diet. This test takes some time, because you have to make sure you've adjusted to a diet without the suspect foods. You give the allergen-free diet at least a few weeks so your body gets used to the missing allergens.

  To determine which foods may be triggers, they're reintroduced one by one with three to four days between each reintroduction. After you start reintroducing the foods, you keep a log or journal of what you've eaten and what, if any, reactions you experienced. After a reaction occurs, you again eliminate that food to see whether the situation reverses — if you broke out in a rash, for example, you make sure the rash goes away.

Be sure to replace any vitamins and other nutrients you'd be getting from a suspect food with something else, either a vitamin supplement or another food source, during the elimination period.

Working within Your Food Limits to Avoid Inflammation

The best way to avoid the inflammatory responses some foods can create is to know your limits and know what you can and can't eat. As you discover throughout this book, many serious health issues — diabetes, heart problems, cancer — can be somewhat managed through food.

The key is knowing which foods are good, which are bad, and which are okay in moderation. Here are some tips to help you live with your sensitivities:

✔ **Pay attention.** Know which foods cause you discomfort and how you'll react to them. Does your stomach make strange noises after you've had a glass of milk? Does red wine make you feel congested? If so, you likely have an intolerance or sensitivity to these items and, depending on the severity of the discomfort, you'll want to either eliminate them from your diet or limit the amount you consume. Read labels carefully to avoid accidental ingestion of the problem food.

✔ **Know your limits and vary your diet.** Sometimes the amount of a particular food creates more problems more than the food itself. Research shows that eating the same thing three or more times in a week can cause stomach distress, so mix up your diet. Really liking salad is okay, but limit it to once or twice a week — or eat different kinds of salads — to avoid issues.

✔ **Find an alternative.** You can almost always find healthy substitutions for the foods on your do-not-eat list; you just have to be open to trying them. Does milk make you bloated or give you intestinal problems? Try almond milk. Have a hankering for some cheese but can't handle what it does to you? Try some goat cheese, which you may tolerate better than cheese made from cow's milk.

✔ **Change your preparation styles.** What if the problem isn't the food but the way you prepare it? Sure, those french fries are great when they come right out of the fryer, but what if you used sweet potatoes instead of white potatoes and then baked them instead of fried them? You'd consume more nutrients without adding trans fats from the oil.

Chapter 3

Determining Inflammation's Role in Chronic Diseases

The body is equipped to take care of itself in many situations, sending signals to create healthy inflammation levels where needed. Catch a cold, and the immune system instantly sends a message to the body to start fighting it off. Twist your ankle while hiking, and the area around it instantly starts to swell, creating a cushioned protection while the injury starts to heal.

Sometimes, however, the body's defense mechanism works against itself, creating problems instead of solving them. Whether the signals get crossed or the process kicks into high gear, the body may fight itself when there's no real reason to engage. The result of this overreaction is chronic illness in the heart, the nerves, the lungs, the joints — just about anywhere.

In this chapter, we examine a variety of chronic illnesses, from heart disease, asthma, and diabetes to obesity and problems with the digestive and immune systems. In addition to helping you gain a better understanding of these illnesses, we identify the role inflammation plays in each of them as well as what you can do to prevent or delay symptoms.

Understanding Chronic Diseases

Chronic diseases are those that aren't communicable; that is, they're not contagious. They're usually long-lasting and don't just go away on their own like a cold or the flu does. Chronic diseases include heart disease, diabetes, cancer, and arthritis — all diseases that invade the body and plan to stay. Most chronic diseases are never cured completely, so your best bet is to avoid getting them in the first place.

The Centers for Disease Control offer some interesting — and frightening — statistics regarding chronic diseases:

- Chronic diseases are responsible for 7 of 10 deaths in the United States each year.
- About 133 million Americans — about half the adults — live with at least one form of chronic illness.
- More than 75 percent of healthcare costs can be attributed to chronic illness.

Inflammation is a common denominator among chronic diseases. Causes of inflammation — such as an inflammatory diet, cigarette smoking, chronic infections, daily stress, nutrient deficiencies, toxins, and lack of exercise — combined with genetic predispositions are a recipe for chronic disease.

Figure 3-1 shows how these factors can lead to systemic inflammation, which can later lead to chronic diseases such as heart and cardiovascular diseases, metabolic diseases (diabetes, obesity, metabolic syndrome), bone disease, and depression. Inflammation leads to low energy and makes you more prone to getting sick and moody, making you less motivated to exercise and further leading to skeletal muscle weakness and more inflammation.

This cycle is self-perpetuating — unless you start to do something about it by changing your diet and lifestyle. Research has shown that dietary and lifestyle changes are more effective than any medication in reducing your risk of chronic disease and can prevent prediabetes from turning into diabetes. Keep in mind that changing your diet to stop inflammation isn't just a temporary fix — it's something you have to commit to following for the rest of your life.

Inflammation may be an underlying cause in multiple disease processes because it interferes with multiple body functions. For example, leaky gut syndrome is a part of the mechanism by which food allergies, sensitivities, intolerances, and toxins play a role in the development of autoimmune diseases.

Autoimmune diseases are chronic diseases in which the body attacks itself through out-of-control inflammation. Besides genetics, dietary factors play a major role in autoimmune diseases. For example, studies have shown that people with certain types of autoimmune diseases, such as Sjögren's disease and Graves' disease, have a greater intolerance to gluten and a higher risk of developing celiac disease.

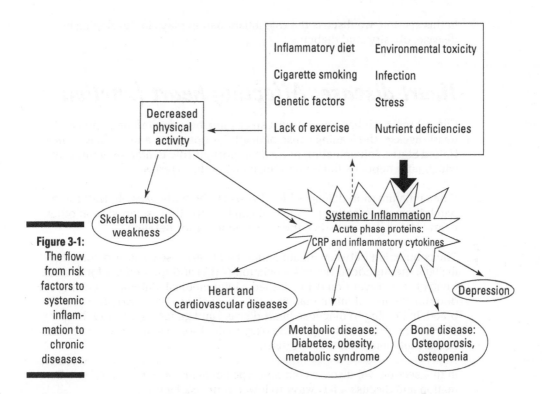

Figure 3-1:
The flow
from risk
factors to
systemic
inflam-
mation to
chronic
diseases.

A naturopathic physician can help identify causes of inflammation and why the body is attacking itself as well as help reduce the symptoms of many chronic diseases. *Naturopathic medicine* puts the focus on holistic medicine and proactive prevention — including good nutrition — and stresses the body's ability to maintain and restore optimal health. Naturopathic physicians can diagnose the same way medical doctors (MDs) do but use natural healing agents. Although naturopathic medicine is a growing practice, naturopaths may still be in short supply in some areas. To find one in your area visit the American Association of Naturopathic Physicians website, www.naturopathic.org.

Connecting Heart Disease, Obesity, and Diabetes to Inflammation

Your body often doesn't take on one disease at a time. Instead, you may get one chronic illness initially, and that illness can lead to others. Obesity, for example, is considered a chronic disease on its own, but it's also a factor in other chronic illnesses such as heart disease and diabetes. You can reduce your risk for all these illnesses by taking inflammatory foods and factors out of your lifestyle.

In this section, we discuss the role inflammation plays in developing heart disease, obesity, and diabetes.

Heart disease: Affecting heart function

Clinical research has uncovered a strong link between inflammation and heart disease, the leading cause of death for both men and women in the United States. Inflammation plays an important role in *atherosclerosis,* in which fatty deposits build up in the lining of the arteries.

When inflammation damages blood vessels, the body uses cholesterol to patch them up, creating plaque that can lead to atherosclerosis and other heart-related diseases. (See the nearby sidebar for details.)

The connection between inflammation and heart disease is so strong that in 2003, the American Heart Association (AHA) and the Centers for Disease Control and Prevention (CDC) issued a joint medical statement opening the door for the use of inflammatory markers, such as C-reactive protein in the blood, in helping to diagnose heart disease and gauge its severity. In other words, the two agencies gave the okay to doctors to start drawing a line connecting inflammation to heart disease.

In this section, we discuss common types of heart disease related to inflammation and discuss a few ways to lower your risk factors.

Looking at common types of heart disease

The types of heart disease range from a minor arrhythmia — irregular heartbeat — to a major heart attack or stroke. Symptoms and causes vary, but each one carries its own risk factors, treatment, and, in many cases, preventive measures to avoid it altogether. Here we take a look at the most common types of heart disease related to inflammation and signs you can look for to identify each one:

- **Cardiovascular disease:** Cardiovascular disease, or *atherosclerosis,* is commonly known as hardening of the arteries. Cardiovascular disease is caused by a buildup of fatty plaques in your arteries which, over time, can make your arteries hard and stiff.

    Major risk factors of cardiovascular disease are smoking, being overweight, lack of exercise, and an unhealthy diet.

- **Coronary artery disease:** Coronary artery disease (CAD) occurs when fatty plaque builds up in the arteries of the heart, and the CDC lists it as the most common form of heart disease in the United States. More than 7 million Americans suffer from coronary artery disease, and an estimated 500,000 Americans die from it each year.

The plaque buildup can lead to *angina,* or chest pain that occurs when the heart doesn't receive enough blood, which can later lead to more serious problems such as heart failure, arrhythmia, or heart attack. Symptoms of coronary artery disease include chest pain or discomfort, shortness of breath, pain in the arms or shoulder, feeling lightheaded or faint, or pain in the jaw, neck, or back.

Patching blood vessels with cholesterol

LDL cholesterol molecules (the bad cholesterol) get oxidized in the blood vessels, leading to the inflammatory reactions that result in clogged arteries.

As the figure below shows, any type of damage to the blood vessel wall — due to infection, high blood pressure, bad food, and so on — gets the immune system involved by telling LDL cholesterol and *monocytes* (a type of white blood cell) to release inflammatory mediators, like CRP, to help address the damage. The monocytes

continue to transform and secrete inflammatory cytokines and reactive oxygen species (ROS), creating more free-radical damage to the blood-vessel cells and more oxidation of the LDLs. This eventually turns into the atherosclerotic plaque that builds up and clogs the arteries, leading to heart attacks and strokes.

Eating a diet rich in antioxidants such as vitamin E prevents the oxidation of the LDL cholesterol molecules that initiates the inflammatory cascade that results in clogging of the arteries.

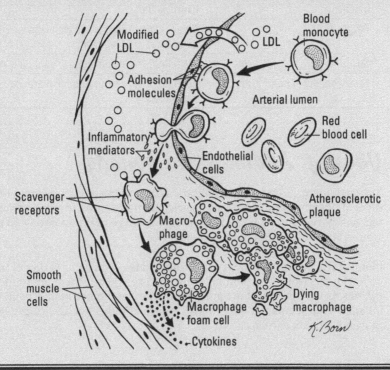

Reducing your risk factors for heart disease

The American Heart Association reports that in 2006, approximately 73,600,000 people had high blood pressure and 17,600,000 had coronary artery disease. Cardiovascular disease caused the deaths of more than 831,200 people in 2006, accounting for more than 34 percent of all deaths that year.

Understanding what those numbers mean and how they relate to you is an important step in taking away the fear of numbers while you tailor your lifestyle to keep you from being a statistic. The best way to do that is to look at the risk factors, compare them to your lifestyle, and make changes to reduce the risks you can control. Table 3-1 lists some of the more common risk factors for heart disease and what you can do to counteract them.

Table 3-1	Risk Factors for Heart Disease
Risk Factor	*What You Can Do to Reduce Your Risk*
Smoking	Quit smoking immediately.
High blood pressure	Eat foods low in saturated fat and sodium.
Obesity	Eliminate refined sugars and processed foods; eat foods low in saturated fat.
Inactivity	Exercise daily.
Poor diet	Replace processed foods with lean meats, vegetables, and legumes.
Stress	Include 30 minutes of yoga in your daily routine.
Family history of heart disease	Eat foods low in saturated fat; increase vegetables.

Obesity: Adding extra pounds

Although many industrialized countries have seen steady increases in the rates of obesity, none have seen as great an increase as the United States: In a ten-year period from 1997 to 2007, the percentage of obese people in the U.S. climbed from 19.4 percent to 26.6 percent.

Blaming the fast-food industry, lack of exercise, or a general diet of overindulgence for the world's expanding waistline is easy, but there are hidden explanations as well. Researchers are finding more and more instances in which inflammation seems not only to prevent weight loss but also to cause people to gain even more weight.

Obesity puts the body into a state of chronic, low-grade inflammation, which is born in the fat cells lying under the skin. When a body is obese, it secretes chemicals called cytokines from the glial cells, which are part of the nervous system. These *cytokines* are molecules that set inflammation into motion. Some of them, interleukin-1 (IL-1) and TFN-alpha, can make you sleepy and irritable. These molecules alert the liver to act immediately, and the liver creates C-reactive protein, which is one sign of inflammation.

White adipose tissue, or fat cells, releases a number of inflammatory chemical signals, called *adipokines,* that affect the body as a whole. The fat cells then become part of the *endocrine system* — the system that regulates growth and reproduction and, when out of balance, increases the risk of insulin resistance, diabetes, heart disease, and other illnesses.

How cortisol release due to stress promotes weight gain

When your body is under stress or your blood contains low levels of hormones called *glucocorticoids*, the pituitary gland in the brain secretes a hormone called *acetylcholinesterase* (ACTH) which signals the adrenal gland on the kidney to secrete cortisol. *Cortisol* is a hormone that increases blood sugar; suppresses the immune system; decreases bone formation; and affects fat, protein, and carbohydrate metabolism, which can lead to weight gain. Cortisol levels are controlled by the part of the brain called the hypothalamus.

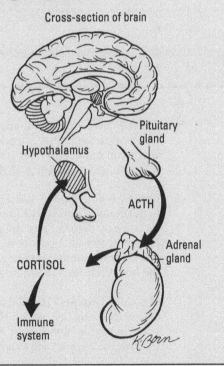

Cross-section of brain

Pituitary gland

Hypothalamus

ACTH

CORTISOL

Adrenal gland

Immune system

Is metabolic syndrome a cause or effect of inflammation?

Metabolic syndrome occurs when a person has a series of metabolic symptoms that, when combined, put the person at an increased risk of coronary heart disease, stroke, and type 2 diabetes. The American Heart Association lists these symptoms as the core group resulting in metabolic syndrome:

- Abdominal obesity (excessive belly fat)
- Elevated triglycerides (blood fat disorders that create plaque buildup)
- High blood pressure
- Insulin resistance/glucose intolerance
- Increased risk and susceptibility to blood clotting
- Inflammatory state (elevated C-reactive protein in the blood)

In metabolic syndrome, the enemy is excessive insulin caused by *insulin resistance,* which creates an imbalance between blood sugar (glucose) and insulin. The cells of the body become resistant to the insulin's attempts to bring the glucose into the cells, and the pancreas produces more insulin to try to make up for this.

Insulin resistance is worsened by inflammatory signals because inflammation does not allow the cells of the body to take in glucose; therefore, sugar levels rise in the blood and can get high enough to cause diabetes. Inflammation kicks in to battle the insulin resistance, creating elevated CRP levels and increasing the risks of stroke and coronary heart disease.

The low-level chronic inflammation of obesity makes your brain and body less responsive to the normal cues (mediated by the adipokines) that signal when you're full and help you to maintain normal body weight. The inflammation also tells your adrenal glands to produce more of the compound cortisol.

Cortisol is your body's natural anti-inflammatory chemical and is produced in high amounts during chronic stress and obesity. Cortisol helps keep energy on track by determining the right type and amount of carbohydrate, fat, or protein that your body needs at any particular time. It moves the body's fat stores from one location to another and prevents the release of substances in the body that lead to inflammation.

Cortisol's response to inflammation is to produce more fat cells around the abdomen (belly fat), which then increases fluid retention, raises blood pressure, increases blood sugar and the risk of insulin resistance, and increases the risks of memory loss and muscle and bone weakness.

Diabetes: Wreaking havoc with your blood sugar

Inflammation and blood sugar have a somewhat tumultuous, circular relationship. When you have high blood sugar, chemicals are released throughout your body, weakening your immune system and kicking inflammation into gear to help protect the body. Because the immune system has been weakened, however, inflammation goes into overdrive and raises the blood sugar, further weakening the immune system.

When you eat, your body breaks down carbohydrates into *glucose,* a simple sugar that travels through your blood and that your muscle cells and other cells take in and use as an energy source. *Insulin* serves as the glucose police in that it regulates how much glucose remains in your blood. When glucose begins to build up, the pancreas (the organ behind the stomach) releases more insulin.

In the ideal situation, the pancreas produces the insulin the body needs, and the body cells respond by taking in sugar. But a condition called *insulin resistance* inhibits the way glucose can get into the body's cells. Inflammation may be behind the poor reception between the cells and the insulin signals. The glucose builds up in the blood, leading to further inflammation and intensifying the problem.

Inflammation from multiple causes increases insulin resistance because the cells become less responsive to the role of insulin in trying to get the glucose into the cell. Likewise, high blood-sugar levels caused by eating too many sweets, empty calories, and simple carbohydrates force the pancreas to produce more insulin to try to clean up the glucose and bring it into the cells. The more you tax your pancreas by eating sugary foods, the more likely your cells will become insulin resistant, increasing your risk for diabetes.

Figure 3-2 shows how inflammation both causes and is caused by insulin resistance. Infection, stress, toxins, genetic factors, and poor diet increase inflammation, which contributes to increased insulin resistance. Insulin resistance leads to decreased glucose metabolism, which leads to high blood sugar and high insulin levels. High blood sugar and insulin levels contribute to weight gain and increased adipose (fat) tissue. High blood sugar, insulin levels, and bad fats contribute to further inflammation by blocking delta-6 desaturase, an enzyme that's important in decreasing inflammation, and enhancing delta-5, an inflammatory enzyme.

The key to stopping the cycle is to find ways to lower the inflammation, which then works to lower the blood sugar levels.

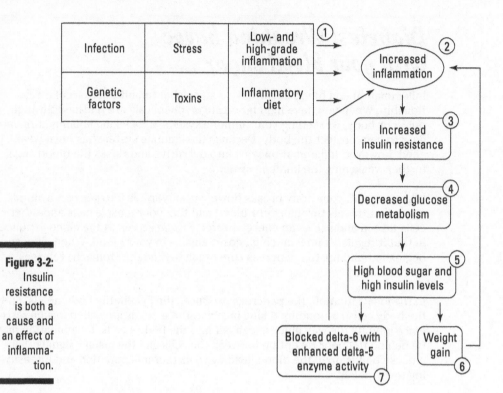

Figure 3-2:
Insulin
resistance
is both a
cause and
an effect of
inflamma-
tion.

Contributing to Cancer

Researchers continue to find connections between cancer and inflammation. For example, medical researchers have found that

- Inflammation can cause DNA changes. A study conducted by the Massachusetts Institute of Technology (MIT) shows a correlation between the DNA damage caused by inflammation and colorectal cancer.

- Recurring infections due to viruses, bacteria, and even overgrowth of yeast can set the body up so it's prone to developing cancer cells. For example, certain strains of HPV (human papillomavirus) increase the risk of developing cervical cancer.

- Toxins in food, like nitrosamines in cured and smoked meats, can stimulate the growth of cancer cells.

- Chronic inflammation helps existing tumors grow and can encourage cancer stem cells to replicate. A study at the University of Michigan's Comprehensive Cancer Center in 2010 suggested that the link between the stem cells of breast cancer and inflammation can promote recurrence of the cancer.

When inflammation persists, it creates a negative environment that can support the development of tumors, and pre-cancerous cells can become malignant. Researchers believe this happens because many of the processes that occur in chronic inflammation can contribute to tumor growth and disease progression.

Inflammation starts with the help of *cytokines* — chemicals that send signals to certain cells to either enhance or suppress the body's immune system. These cytokines are proteins whose primary responsibility is to attack foreign bodies or damaged cells or to signal other parts of the immune system to get in gear and attack. Cancer cells are just the type of cells cytokines should be attacking. However, although cancer cells have somehow lost their ability to control their own growth, they're otherwise normal, healthy cells. Because of this, the immune system doesn't recognize these cells as foreign, so it doesn't attack.

Asthma: Inflaming the Lungs

Inflammation plays an important role in the everyday functioning of the lungs. Think of all the bacteria, viruses, dust, and everything else floating through the air, and then think of yourself breathing it in. Small amounts of inflammation are at work throughout the day battling these particles, creating and using an antibody called *immunoglobulin E* (IgE) to aid in breaking down the pollutants.

The lungs of people with asthma, however, overreact to these particles. The immune system mass-produces the IgE antibodies, which then attach to something called *mast cells.* Each time someone with asthma inhales the offending particles, the antibodies lock onto the invaders and cause the mast cells to release histamine and leukotrienes, which irritate the lining of the airways. The irritation causes the airways to spasm and constrict, making breathing difficult; the harder the person tries to breathe, the more irritated and constricted the airways become.

Atopy, or IgE reactions, is the greatest predisposing factor to developing asthma. Many people with asthma also have sensitivity to sulfites, which are found in certain foods and are used in wine-making and preserving dried fruit.

Asthma can be caused by a variety of factors that result in airway inflammation, and triggers for asthma attacks may be allergic or nonallergic. Allergic asthma, or *extrinsic* asthma, is triggered by allergens. Nonallergic asthma, or *intrinsic* asthma, can be triggered by anything but is not considered an allergic reaction.

Allergic triggers include the following:

- ✔ Cat or dog hair and saliva
- ✔ Dust mites, mold, or spores
- ✔ Pollen

Nonallergic triggers include the following:

- ✔ Smoke, smog, fumes
- ✔ Natural gas, cooking fuel
- ✔ Exercise
- ✔ Viral respiratory infections
- ✔ Weather changes, such as exposure to cold air

Disrupting Your Digestive System

Inflammation steps in when the digestive tract goes askew, whether it's because something has physically injured the tract or you've eaten your way to trouble. Sometimes the inflammation takes the form of a mild stomach issue such as diarrhea or constipation, and other times it can lead to something much more serious.

Crohn's disease and ulcerative colitis are forms of *inflammatory bowel disease* (IBD), which are inflammation-related diseases that affect the colon and small intestines. In both conditions, parts of the digestive tract — also known as the gastrointestinal (GI) tract — become inflamed and create problems with digestion:

- ✔ **Crohn's disease:** *Crohn's disease* causes inflammation anywhere along the GI tract and can spread into the layers of bowel tissue. It can cause inflammation in several areas of the tract at once, leaving healthy bowel trapped between two segments of diseased bowel.

  Researchers believe Crohn's disease is a result of the body's immune system creating an inflammatory response to misidentified invaders, building a protective area against certain foods. What results is abdominal pain and diarrhea as the body attempts to rid itself of the invaders. Other symptoms of Crohn's disease include rectal bleeding, weight loss, fatigue, skin irritations, and fever. Bleeding can become excessive, leading to anemia (low iron).

✓ **Ulcerative colitis:** *Ulcerative colitis* creates inflammation and ulcers only in the top layer of the lining of the large intestine, and it often affects the rectum. Symptoms of ulcerative colitis are very similar to those of Crohn's disease, causing some confusion in trying to establish a diagnosis between the two. The symptoms include anemia, fatigue, weight loss, loss of appetite, bloody diarrhea mixed with mucus, loss of body fluids and nutrients, skin lesions, joint pain and stunted growth (especially in children), and abdominal pain.

Medications can ease some of the discomfort of inflammatory bowel disorders, and surgery is necessary for about two-thirds of people with Crohn's disease.

Inflammation of the digestive tract can cause further problems in other parts of the body, too. *Leaky gut syndrome* is a phenomenon whereby the cells of the digestive tract are inflamed and no longer provide a protective barrier between the inside and outside worlds of your digestive tract. It also can make you feel bloated and fatigued, especially after eating.

The first step to treating IBD is to identify the causes of inflammation — diet, stressors, nutrient deficiencies, genetic susceptibility, and so on. Next, remove the inflammatory foods from your diet. You also have to heal the gut, which may involve taking anti-inflammatory drugs and supplements such as omega-3 fatty acids and l-glutamine. The inflamed gut is unable to absorb vitamins such as B12, so after healing, you can then address nutrient deficiencies.

Knocking Your Immune System Off-kilter

The body's immune system is a wonderful thing when it's working properly. It keeps infection at bay and protects an injured area from getting reinjured while it heals. Sometimes, however, the immune system misfires and sends out signals when none are needed. In those instances, the inflammation attacks the body, creating *autoimmune disorders* such as lupus, rheumatoid arthritis, and multiple sclerosis. We discuss these autoimmune disorders in this section.

Autoimmune disorders seem to be associated with leaky gut syndrome (see the preceding section), and people with these disorders also have a higher incidence of vitamin D deficiency. An anti-inflammatory diet and stress reduction may improve autoimmune conditions.

Getting to know lupus

Systemic lupus erythematosus (SLE) is an autoimmune disorder that affects the kidneys and other organs as well as the skin and joints.

Lupus appears to be a women's disease for the most part — more than 90 percent of those diagnosed are women between the ages of 15 and 40. People with relatives who have lupus have a 5 to 13 percent chance of developing the disease, although people whose mothers have lupus have just a 5 percent chance of getting it. In most cases, people diagnosed with lupus have a relative who has been diagnosed with some other autoimmune disease.

Although lupus is largely a genetic disorder, some environmental factors can trigger the illness: exposure to ultraviolet sun rays or rays from fluorescent bulbs, sulfa drugs, penicillin, an infection, a cold or other viral infection, exhaustion, stress, or an injury.

The severity of SLE can range widely; it can be very mild, or it can turn fatal. Symptoms of SLE vary according to which part of the body is affected:

- **Brain and nervous system:** Symptoms may include headaches, personality changes, psychotic episodes, tingling in the arms and legs, and seizures.

- **Digestive tract:** Symptoms may include nausea, vomiting, and abdominal pain.

- **Kidneys:** Look for discolored urine.

- **Heart:** Symptoms include arrhythmia.

- **Lungs:** Symptoms include coughing up blood.

- **Skin:** Skin rashes, particularly on the face, appear if SLE is affecting the skin.

Some common symptoms, regardless of where SLE attacks, are fatigue, weight loss, unexplained fever, sores in the mouth, and hair loss.

There's no cure for SLE, but you can control the symptoms. Dietary changes are one way to help relieve some of the pain and discomfort. Some medications alleviate discomfort for some varieties of SLE, and corticosteroid creams are used for skin rashes.

Arthritis: Making your joints ache

The word *arthritis* literally means "inflammation of the joints." Most forms of arthritis are *autoimmune diseases,* a result of a misinformed attack by the immune system on part of the body. Some of the more common forms of arthritis caused by inflammation are

- ✔ Rheumatoid arthritis
- ✔ Gout
- ✔ Systemic lupus erythematosis
- ✔ Degenerative joint disease

Some of the symptoms of inflammation associated with arthritis are redness, joint pain, warm swollen areas, and limited ability to bend the joints.

Research has shown that certain foods, such as those in the nightshade or *Solonacea* family (potatoes, tomatoes, eggplant, bell peppers) contribute to inflammation in rheumatoid arthritis (RA) and osteoarthritis (OA) for some people. About 10 percent of people have sensitivities or allergies to the nightshade family and, as with any sensitivity, this situation can increase the risk of arthritis. Anti-inflammatory foods such as fish oil help reduce the inflammation of RA and OA.

Looking at osteoarthritis

In *osteoarthritis,* inflammation of the joint compresses the nerves and causes the shock-absorbing system between the joints to degenerate. Osteoarthritis is also known as *age-related arthritis,* and with good reason: It affects more than 70 percent of adults between the ages of 55 and 78. The majority of those affected are women.

Osteoarthritis may also be caused by obesity or long-term overuse of a joint during work or in sports. Repeated motion and injuries contribute to the inflammatory process in arthritis. For example, a football player who injures himself is more susceptible to arthritis in the affected area. A joint injury at a younger age can mean osteoarthritis later.

Although osteoarthritis isn't curable, you can manage its pain and other symptoms. Some doctors advise taking acetaminophen for pain, and lifestyle changes may also relieve some of the tenderness. Exercise helps keep the joints moving and can help with weight loss, particularly if that's relevant to the osteoarthritis. (We cover exercises to mitigate inflammation in Chapter 19.)

Experts also recommend getting plenty of rest, keeping the joints protected, and eating a healthy, well-balanced diet. Part of that includes drinking enough water to keep the joints and the rest of the body hydrated.

Recognizing rheumatoid arthritis

Rheumatoid arthritis (RA) is an autoimmune disease that causes inflammation in the lining of the smaller joints in the hands and feet, often leading to bone deterioration and joint deformity. Some sufferers experience intermittent flare-ups, and others see the symptoms and pain go into a remission-like dormancy for long periods of time.

More than 1.3 million Americans suffer from RA — about 1 percent of the country's population. It occurs two or three times as often in women as it does in men and generally occurs between the ages of 30 and 60, although it can occur in teens and even children.

No one knows the cause of RA, although researchers have a list of suspects; some believe it's triggered by an infectious bacteria or virus, and others think it may be linked to a female hormone, resulting in the high differential between the number of women who develop RA over men. Many researchers believe smoking plays a role as well, at least by weakening the body's immune system.

Diagnosis includes checking for inflammation in the blood with tests such as the C-reactive protein (CRP) test and radiological studies. Approximately 75 percent of people test positive for the rheumatoid factor (RF) antibody in their blood, which may lead to RA. Having RF show up on a blood test doesn't necessarily mean you have it, nor does not having RF mean you don't, because about 20 percent of tests result in false positives and false negatives. Your doctor will take into account your clinical symptoms combined with these tests to determine your diagnosis.

Rheumatoid arthritis is a chronic disease, but it's manageable. Doctors may prescribe certain medications to relieve the pain of rheumatoid arthritis, but people with RA can also do many things at home without medication. Applying heat and cold to the affected area can alleviate some of the pain, and exercising regularly helps keep bones and joints moving, reducing the risk of stiffness.

Following an anti-inflammatory diet and avoiding the nightshade family can aid in reducing the pain and inflammation of RA. Tobacco is also in the nightshade family, so avoid smoking as well.

Nerve attacks: Linking inflammation to multiple sclerosis

Multiple sclerosis (MS) is an autoimmune disorder that showcases how violent the human body can be when it turns on itself. With multiple sclerosis, the body's immune system eats away at the protective covering that envelops the nerves, interfering with communication between the nerves and the brain and eventually leading to degeneration of the nerves themselves. The process MS follows is irreversible. There's no cure, but treatment can lessen the severity of the attacks.

Multiple sclerosis may be difficult to diagnose in the early stages because symptoms tend to come and go, often not resurfacing for months. Symptoms also vary greatly; they may include numbness or tingling in the arms and legs, partial or complete loss of vision, double vision or blurred vision, fatigue, dizziness, and electric shock-type sensations that occur when the head is moved in a certain way. In the most severe cases, people lose the ability to walk or talk.

MS tends to occur in women twice as often as in men, and it's typically diagnosed in people between the ages of 20 and 40. If a member of your family has MS, you have a 1 to 3 percent chance of inheriting the disease. Caucasians whose families originated in northern Europe are at greater risk.

Here are several things you can do at home to relieve the symptoms of multiple sclerosis:

- ✔ **Cool down.** Multiple sclerosis symptoms tend to flare up when your body temperature rises. Try taking a cool bath to bring your temperature back down.

- ✔ **Get plenty of rest.** Fatigue is a common symptom, and getting rest can help you feel better.

- ✔ **Exercise.** Keeping active with mild aerobic exercise helps build strength and muscle coordination if you have mild to moderate MS.

- ✔ **Watch your diet.** Researchers believe multiple sclerosis is an autoimmune disorder caused by inflammation, so look for anti-inflammatory foods.

Part II
Understanding Anti-Inflammatory Nutrition

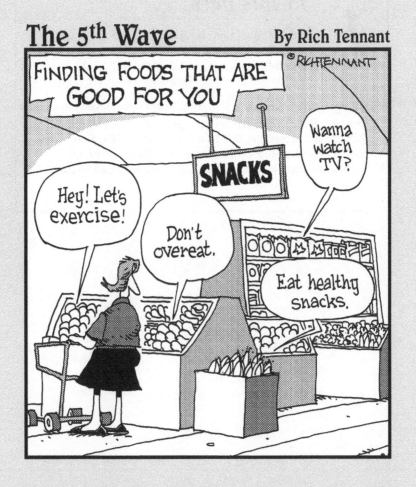

The 5th Wave   By Rich Tennant

FINDING FOODS THAT ARE GOOD FOR YOU

SNACKS

Hey! Let's exercise!

Don't overeat.

Wanna watch TV?

Eat healthy snacks.

In this part . . .

In this part, we talk about food — the good, the bad, and the ugly. We modify the traditional food pyramid to make it anti-inflammatory, and then we take you through the different levels and explain why some foods are better than others. We look at fats, carbohydrates, and proteins, helping you find the good in each as well as the bad. We examine the effects each of these has on inflammation and the link to chronic illness. We also indulge the sweet tooth, because as with most things, treats are good in moderation. Here, we lead you to the best of the best.

Chapter 4

Filling Your Plate to Fight Inflammation

. . . .

In This Chapter

▶ Knowing which foods are good or bad

▶ Making an anti-inflammatory food pyramid

▶ Understanding inflammation factor ratings

. . . .

Almost everyone these days seems to have some understanding of the basic food pyramid: fruits, vegetables, grains, dairy, and meat. Making sure you get the proper number of servings of each group has been a nutritional mainstay in the United States since the early 1990s, and it's spilled over to other countries, as well.

For people fighting inflammation, not only can following the basic food guidelines be inadequate, but it can also aid inflammation, contributing to problems such as diabetes, heart disease, and even certain cancers. Figuring out which foods help in the battle against inflammation and knowing how much of each food you need is a great start to changing to an anti-inflammatory lifestyle that can not only improve how you feel now but also help you make great strides in overall health.

This chapter guides you through the basic food pyramid — and the USDA's new plate image — and the best adjustments you can make to change your menu from one that aids in inflammation to one that fights it.

An anti-inflammatory diet is not designed to help you lose weight (although weight loss is a good possibility because inflammation influences your weight), nor is this diet something that you should consider temporary. Committing to an anti-inflammatory diet is telling yourself that you want to do what you can to get and stay healthy.

Following Recommendations for Good and Bad Food Categories

The food recommendations for an anti-inflammation diet are geared toward keeping your body healthy. These recommendations steer you toward (or away from) both specific foods and general types of foods, so you can design your own menu based on what you know.

Here are some good-food categories to keep in mind when changing to an anti-inflammatory diet:

- ✔ **Omega-3 fatty acids:** You can find these fats, which can help reduce inflammation, in coldwater oily fish, walnuts, flaxseeds, and olive oil. None of those sound appealing? Omega-3 fatty acids are available in supplement form as well.

- ✔ **Protein:** Protein helps build healthy tissues and keeps inflammation at bay. This is where your lean poultry, fish, nuts, and legumes fit in. Protein sources that are high in fiber and nutrients, like legumes, help to decrease inflammation by balancing blood sugar, providing the building blocks to build muscle, and giving you long-term energy.

- ✔ **Fiber:** Here's where your fruits and vegetables, as well as whole grains, come into play. All these foods are rich in fiber, which helps your body fight inflammation. Good news for pasta-lovers is that brown rice pasta makes the list of good-for-you fibers.

- ✔ **Water:** Although your body gets some water in the form of fruits and vegetables, drinking plenty of water every day is still a great idea. Don't like plain water? Use it to make herbal teas or find fruit juices that are 100 percent juice and dilute them with water to keep the sugar concentrations down.

Here are some bad-food categories to avoid when changing to an anti-inflammatory diet:

- ✔ **Sugars:** Researchers have found that sugar increases the risk of obesity, inflammation, and diabetes. Look instead for natural sweeteners, such as honey, agave nectar, pure maple syrup, brown rice syrup, or stevia. For information on sugars and sweeteners, turn to Chapter 8.

- ✔ **Omega-6 fatty acids:** Many of the most common cooking oils are high in omega-6 fatty acids, and diets high in these fats are inflammatory and can lead to increased risks of cancer and heart disease. Reach for the extra-virgin olive oil and the other oils we mention in Chapters 5 and 16.

✔ **Trans fats:** Trans fats, which for a long time appeared in most fast foods, fried foods, and commercial baked goods, do the opposite of what they should: They lower the good cholesterol and raise the bad cholesterol, increasing the risks of obesity and insulin resistance. Many food producers have reformulated recipes so trans fats aren't as plentiful, but these bad fats are still out there, so be sure to read food labels carefully.

✔ **Dairy products:** More than half of the U.S. population has some degree of lactose intolerance and sensitivity to all or some dairy products. This sensitivity can lead to poor digestion, diarrhea, constipation, and stomach distress.

✔ **Meats:** Particularly avoid meats from feedlot-fed animals, red meats, and processed meats, which you find in most supermarkets and restaurants. These meats are high in omega-6 fatty acids, and processed meats have been smoked, cured, or otherwise treated with chemicals. Smoking meats creates nitrosamines, which have been linked to intestinal and breast cancer. Curing isn't as bad unless it involves using preservatives, but it may involve soaking in a salt brine.

✔ **Refined or enriched grains:** Most of the grains found on store shelves or used in baked goods have been stripped of the plant's bulk, which contains the nutritional properties. Refined grains are more powdery and less coarse, and they can speed up the development of cancer and heart disease.

Adapting General Food Recommendations for Your Needs

The food pyramid Americans have come to know — which the United States Department of Agriculture (USDA) introduced in 1992 and revised in 2005 — has long been a symbol of healthy eating and maintaining balance. It offered guidelines for people to follow a balanced menu incorporating foods from each of five groups — fruits, vegetables, grains, meat, and milk — with limited amounts of fats, oils, and sweets.

The USDA acknowledged the pyramid's shortcomings and in June 2011 did away with the pyramid, replacing it with a simplified symbol of a divided plate. The new plate is divided into portions indicating areas for fruits, vegetables, grains, protein (replacing the meat group), and dairy. Fruits and vegetables take up half of the plate, and grains and protein share the other half. Dairy is located where a glass would be on a place setting.

What the food guidelines still don't do is address the individual needs of people fighting inflammation or people trying to stave off diabetes or cancer or heart ailments. How can whole grains and pasta hurt you if you're fighting inflammation? Is having red meat every day a good idea? Are there dangers in certain fruits and vegetables?

In this section, we transform the traditional food pyramid, identifying which foods don't fit with an anti-inflammatory diet, which foods to add, and how to make a new anti-inflammatory pyramid that works for you. We also discuss the new USDA recommendations and the agency's new food plate for nutrition, identifying how it differs from the iconic food pyramid and why we stick with the pyramid to present anti-inflammatory recommendations.

Herbs and spices: Going beyond the five food groups

The USDA's food pyramid and plate stress the importance of getting something from each of the five food groups. They even recommend how much of each you should eat. But the guidelines stop with these food categories. Other foods, spices, and extras should be a part of your diet as you're fighting inflammation or inflammation-related issues.

Many herbs and spices offer many benefits because they contain phytochemicals (the compounds produced by plants), bioflavonoids (the antioxidants found in fruits and vegetables), omega-3 fatty acids, and other antiinflammatory nutrients that enhance the natural foods from the food pyramid.

Here are some of the top anti-inflammatory herbs and spices and what they can do:

- **Cayenne pepper:** Works to kill some cancer cells and clean out the arteries
- **Cumin:** Helps flush toxins from the body and prevents and fights cancers
- **Garlic:** Is anti-inflammatory because of its high sulfur content and has antiviral and antibacterial properties as well
- **Ginger:** Also helps with inflammations causing joint pain (it's a good natural way to beat headaches, too!)
- **Turmeric:** Helps relieve arthritis, tendonitis, and even some autoimmune disorders

Other herbs and spices that aid in the fight against inflammation are black pepper, cinnamon, rosemary, basil, cardamom, chives, cilantro, cloves, and parsley.

When adding herbs and spices to a favorite food, stick to the serving size of about ½ to 1 teaspoon to get the optimum effect. When using fresh herbs, you can be a bit more generous, using roughly twice as much fresh as you would use dried. With fresh ginger, use at least a 1-inch piece to get worthwhile medicinal benefits. Both dried and fresh herbs and spices have great anti-inflammatory benefits.

Creating the anti-inflammatory food pyramid

The common food pyramid offers guidelines for the number of servings a "normal" person should have in terms of fruits, vegetables, milk, meats and beans, and grains. The new plate identifies the food groups — replacing meats with proteins — but doesn't identify how much of each you should have. The new plate even provides altered menus for those with special needs, such as pregnant and breastfeeding women, preschoolers, and people pursuing weight loss.

What the plate *doesn't* do, however, is take into account people whose diets are limited by sensitivities, allergies, or chronic inflammation. Not everyone can tolerate dairy products or grains, and people fighting inflammation likely won't be reaching for red meats or certain vegetables and fruits.

Some foods are more likely than others to be associated with sensitivities, creating even more problems for the body. For example, wheat and dairy can create problems even for people not suffering from celiac disease or lactose intolerance, and corn, eggs, and citrus fruits can cause heightened sensitivities as well. Additionally, eating the same thing too many times in a short time frame, such as a week, can lead to sensitization to the food, and the body may start attacking what is normally a "good" food, thinking it's something foreign.

We've taken the traditional food pyramid and altered it to address just those issues, specifying the inclusion of gluten-free grains, providing alternatives to dairy, and identifying meats and proteins other than red meats.

Getting the full benefits of an anti-inflammatory diet means knowing just how much is enough and then following through. Striking the right nutritional balance is just as important as knowing which foods to eat. For the most part, if you play by the anti-inflammatory rules at least 90 percent of the time, you'll still feel optimum benefits of fighting inflammation.

Need something to help you know what to eat and how much of it to eat? That's what the anti-inflammatory food pyramid is for. See Figure 4-1.

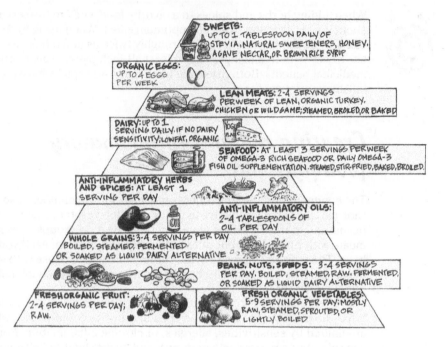

Figure 4-1:
The anti-inflammatory food pyramid.

Table 4-1 contains some tips for making the pyramid.

Table 4-1	Top Recommendations for Each Food Group
Food Group	*What to Select, How to Prepare It, and More*
Water	Drink at least eight glasses of purified or spring water per day.
Fresh organic vegetables	Load up on leafy greens, onions, garlic, and mushrooms. Eat vegetables mostly raw, steamed, sprouted, or lightly boiled; eat a wide range of colors both raw and cooked. Lower glycemic-index vegetables are important for people with a higher risk for developing diabetes, or with metabolic syndrome, prediabetes, and diabetes.
Fresh organic fruit	Top choices include berries (blueberries, raspberries, cherries), pomegranates, and fruits with high antioxidant values.
Vegetable protein	Beans, legumes, lentils, nuts, and seeds fill this category. Top choices are walnuts (omega-3s), almonds, and flaxseeds (omega-3s). Combine beans with whole grains for a complete protein.
Whole grains	Opt for quinoa, brown rice, barley, and steel-cut oats.

Food Group	What to Select, How to Prepare It, and More
Anti-inflammatory oils	Good choices include extra-virgin olive oil, walnut oil, avocado oil, coconut oil, high-oleic sunflower oil, high-oleic safflower oil, and flaxseed oil.
Anti-inflammatory spices	Ginger, turmeric, and garlic are especially good choices.
Seafood and freshwater fish	Sardines, salmon, halibut, and mackerel are the best choices because of their omega-3s. Find recommendations on how to choose lower mercury seafood at `www.vital choice.com`.
Organic dairy products	If you don't have dairy sensitivities, choose fermented dairy products (yogurt, kefir) with live cultures.
Meats	Stick to lean meats, such as poultry (turkey, chicken) and wild game; choose lean cuts, and prepare them mostly by steaming, baking, or broiling.
Free-range organic eggs	Eggs are best for you when they're soft-boiled or poached rather than fried.
Sweets	Sweeten foods using natural sweeteners or eat dark chocolate with at least 70 percent cocoa.

The new food plate is similar to the anti-inflammatory diet in that half the plate is vegetables and fruit, which coincides with getting 5–9 servings of vegetables and 2–4 servings of fruit a day. The other part of the plate is protein and grains. We discuss in this book the importance of eating whole grains rather than refined grains and what types of protein will be anti-inflammatory (such as vegetable protein, omega-3-rich fish, and grass-fed, free-range organic animal protein in moderation). You can replace the dairy in the upper right corner of the food plate with dairy alternatives, such as rice milk or almond milk if you don't tolerate dairy products, or your daily serving of lowfat plain yogurt or unprocessed cheese if you don't have a dairy sensitivity. We also add in anti-inflammatory herbs and spices, fermented foods, and include information on how to prepare food to keep inflammation at bay.

How Foods Stack Up Based on Inflammation Factors

Researchers at the University of South Carolina and the University of Massachusetts created an *inflammation index* in 2009 in an effort to see just how inflammatory peoples' diets really are. After examining nearly 60 years' worth of reports, studies, and articles on foods and how their individual compounds can affect the body, researchers scored foods according to whether they were anti-inflammatory or inflammatory — that is, whether they helped to prevent or alleviate inflammation or whether they were part of the problem.

Researchers then gave each food an *inflammation factor* (IF) rating based on whether it was anti-inflammatory. Foods with positive IF ratings are considered anti-inflammatory, and foods with negative ratings contribute to the development of inflammation.

The formula used to determine each food's IF rating takes into consideration more than 20 factors, including the type and amount of fat in each food, the levels of vitamins and other nutrients, and any anti-inflammatory compounds that may be present. Each food carries the same IF rating for everyone, but your body is going to react to each food differently.

Want to know whether that grapefruit you're eating in the morning is better than a plain bagel with cream cheese? Check out the nutritional breakdown feature on `http://nutritiondata.self.com`. Just enter a food item into the search box at the top of the home page and click Search to see its IF rating and other nutritional info. That grapefruit has an IF rating of 18, and the bagel and cream cheese gets a –640!

Researchers also set a target daily IF value, providing the opportunity to balance anti- and inflammatory foods. The goal of the IF rating is to end the day with an IF score of at least 50, but that doesn't mean you need to, or even should, avoid foods with negative IF ratings. Instead, use the rating system as a tool for balance: If you're not lactose intolerant, it's okay to have a cup of plain yogurt, even though it has an IF rating of –71. Balance that yogurt out with a small spinach salad with olive oil for lunch (one cup of raw spinach has an IF rating of 78 and a teaspoon of olive oil scores 24, for a total of 102). By the end of lunch, your net IF score is 31.

In the following sections, we identify which foods are more inflammatory than others, and which you should be adding to your diet. We list possible problems with various kinds of foods and how likely it is that you may find yourself experiencing some of these issues.

Steering clear of inflammatory foods

Although splurging every once in a while is okay, certain foods are highly inflammatory and should really be avoided. Such foods include high-omega-6 oils (such as those made from corn, safflower, sunflower, and cottonseed), inflammatory saturated fats from animal sources (as found in processed meats like bologna and hot dogs), and refined sugars and trans fats. Minimize or eliminate the amount of processed food and fast food you eat. Many of these foods are high in starch and sugars, as well as refined flours. For people with certain allergies or sensitivities, gluten products (wheat, barley, and rye), soy products, corn and corn products, and foods in the nightshade family (potatoes, tomatoes, and eggplant) can be highly inflammatory.

Here are some of the more common inflammatory foods to avoid and their IF ratings:

- **Breads, rolls, bagels, pancakes, waffles:** –4 to –51
- **Baked goods including cookies, cakes, doughnuts, and muffins:** –107 to –300
- **Cereals (except old-fashioned oatmeal):** –121 to –200
- **Corn syrup:** –63 per teaspoon to –1,100 per cup
- **Crackers, tortillas:** –170
- **Fruit juices, soda:** –50
- **Fried foods:** –80 to –200
- **Hard cheeses, particularly nonorganic:** –120
- **Ice cream and frozen yogurt:** –84 to –157 (frozen yogurt is actually worse)
- **Jams and jellies:** –65
- **Pasta made with white flour:** –57
- **Potatoes:** –88

The easiest way to determine whether a food is going to work for you or against you — whether it's anti-inflammatory or inflammatory — is to simply look at the food and its label. The less "natural" a food seems to be, the higher the possibility that it's going to be inflammatory.

In the ingredients list, look for words like *refined, enriched,* and *processed* — all words that let you know something has been done to the food or the ingredients to make it as it is now. *Refined sugars,* for example, means the product has been stripped of everything but the chemical compound sucrose, so all the plant's nutritional elements are lost.

In some cases, using organic or natural products in place of those that are more commercially produced can improve the food's inflammation factor, but sometimes it's just best to do without the food altogether.

Knowing which foods are inflammatory can be as simple as keeping one rule of thumb in mind: If it doesn't look like it did originally, it's probably inflammatory. For example, whole grains, such as bulgur wheat, brown rice, and oats, all look like they do in the wild: complete with the germ and the entire grain kernel. After those grains become refined, they take on an entirely different appearance. For example, refined brown rice becomes starchy white rice.

That's not to say that you have to eat everything raw. You can change a food's appearance on your own, after you have it in the kitchen: Food can be cut, crushed, steamed, and so on. Chapter 16 gives you advice on making your home cooking endeavors less inflammatory.

Hailing the anti-inflammatory foods

The good news is that there are plenty of good foods that can help prevent or lessen inflammation. *Anti-inflammatory foods* are those that make you feel better and reduce your risk of inflammation and chronic disease. Whole, natural foods top the list. Processed meats and most red meats are no-nos, but lean poultry, fish, and even some red meat such as venison and bison go a long way in fighting inflammation.

Most fruits and vegetables, particularly those grown organically and eaten fresh rather than canned, pass the muster on the list of anti-inflammatory foods. They're just naturally good for you. The following sections highlight some anti-inflammatory foods and their IF ratings.

Onions

Like garlic, onions have high sulfur content. They also have antiviral and antibacterial properties. The World Health Organization (WHO) recognizes the health benefits of onions and supports their use in the treatment of atherosclerosis (hardened arteries). Onions are rich in fructooligosaccharides, which are very beneficial in colon health. One cup of diced raw onions has an IF rating of 374, and one tablespoon has a rating of 23.

Mushrooms

Mushrooms are anti-inflammatory. Most edible mushrooms are full of proteins, beneficial vitamins and minerals, and antioxidants and amino acids. They also contain polysaccharides (complex carbohydrates) that are good for the immune system. The most beneficial edible mushrooms are the Asian, maitake, oyster, and shiitake mushrooms. These mushrooms should be eaten cooked, not raw.

Mushrooms have a small negative IF rating — maitake mushrooms, for example, have an IF rating of –9 for one cup — but their other health benefits outweigh that rating.

On their own, mushrooms provide good protein with zero cholesterol and fats; some mushrooms can help to lower cholesterol levels. The beta-glucans and linoleic acid levels have anti-carcinogen benefits, helping battle breast and prostate cancer. Mushrooms are also rich in calcium, vitamin D, iron, potassium, and selenium, so they help lower blood pressure and fight anemia while helping to strengthen bones. The first statins discovered were found in medicinal molds, and the oyster mushroom naturally contains a statin.

Fermented foods

Fermented foods — those that microorganisms have partially broken down — are strong fighters against inflammation because they still contain the good bacteria, yeast, or mold that many processing practices kill off. Fermented foods include cheese, miso, kimchi, yogurt, sauerkraut, vinegar, sour cream, olives, and pickles.

The IF ratings for fermented foods vary; for example, sauerkraut and vinegar are slightly anti-inflammatory, while miso and sour cream are mildly to strongly inflammatory. There is no standard for this food category, but you can find the ratings for each food at http://nutritiondata.self.com.

Fermented foods are easier to digest (although fermented dairy products should be avoided if you have dairy sensitivities). They also aid in absorption of certain nutrients and enzymes within the fermented foods.

Implementing the Plan

At first glance, changing your diet to be anti-inflammatory may seem intimidating, maybe even a little frightening. But look at this change as a new beginning — a new start for a healthy lifestyle that will make you feel better. Don't view this diet as a list of restrictions. Instead, view it as a challenge. Give yourself small goals: "This week I plan to go without cheese." Or "I'll add a serving of nuts or seeds to my diet each day this week."

In Chapter 16, you can find tips for cleaning out your kitchen and restocking it with the foods and spices that best serve an anti-inflammatory diet. The temptation to eat something bad is much weaker when the bad food isn't there, just as inspiration to eat better comes more easily when the good food is staring you in the face.

Your routine will change, too. Instead of spending time and money sitting in the drive-through lane of that fast food joint you pass on your way home at night, you'll be in the kitchen cooking, and you'll know exactly what you're eating (no mystery ingredients!). To make it more fun, turn meal preparations into a family activity and get everyone to pitch in. If you get stuck for ideas, turn to Part III for recipes from breakfast to snacks to evening entertaining.

Chapter 5

Feeling the Love (or Hate) in Fats

....

....

For years you've been told to avoid fats, go for lean meats, stay away from this, never eat that. But what if someone were to tell you that fat is not only good for you but necessary? Although too much dietary fat can be bad, fat is one of three macronutrients — along with protein and carbohydrates — that turn into energy for your body, helping it get through its day-to-day functions. In fact, of the three macronutrients, dietary fat has more food energy per mass than carbohydrates and protein, making it an excellent form of stored energy for the body.

Fat also supports some of your body's functions — lubricating body surfaces; insulating from cold; promoting strong brain function; carrying fat-soluble vitamins A, D, E, and K; and cell signaling as part of the endocrine system, to name a few. Cholesterol, which your liver makes from saturated fat, serves as the base for estrogen, cortisone, and testosterone, and without the right amount, your body doesn't make enough of these hormones. Therefore, fat is a vital part of your health.

Of course, not all fats are created equal. The trick is to get the right kinds of dietary fat in the right amounts. In this chapter, we introduce the good fats and note why they're so good, talk about the bad fats and what makes them bad, and note some easy ways to tell the difference.

Getting the Message: Fat, Inflammation, and Cell Signals

Fat cells aren't just the building blocks of obesity. Fat helps the body absorb nutrients, maintains the integrity of cell membranes, and even keeps transmission lines between nerve cells open. Here are some ways fat contributes to the signaling systems in the body:

- **Insulating nerves:** Nerve cells, or neurons, are covered by a fatty *myelin sheath* that insulates and protects the electrical signals from interference. Nerve cells are more efficient at signaling when they're coated with fat, allowing the brain to run faster and create better connections. Getting enough of the good dietary fats during pregnancy helps boost the child's intelligence.

- **Controlling what goes in and out of cells:** Good fats get incorporated into the membrane of every cell in your body. A lot of cell-to-cell communication occurs on the *cell membrane,* the outer covering of the cell, so the fats you ingest can positively or negatively affect cell-to-cell communication.

- **Serving as raw materials for making hormones and other chemicals:** Fatty acids are part of the structure of chemical messengers such as sex hormones and *prostaglandins,* a hormone-like chemical that kind of calls the shots on many of the body's functions — including inflammatory responses.

- **Sending out signals:** Together, fat cells in the lower belly area may act as an organ that sends chemical signals to the rest of the body — signals that may trigger heart attacks, cancer, and other diseases.

Good fats like those from fish oils and walnuts help fat cells send the right types of signals to the body. But when you get too much fat — or the wrong kind of fat — things start to go awry. Eating hydrogenated fats and fat-soluble toxins sends the signals out of balance and affects your *endocrine system,* the system that regulates hormones and metabolism.

Exploring Different Kinds of Fat

Fat got a bad rap around the end of the 20th century. The wrong fats, or even too much of the good fats, can open the doors to a laundry list of illnesses. However, cutting out fat entirely is a mistake, because good fats do exist.

Knowing which fats are good for you and which ones you should avoid can help keep inflammation and therefore chronic illness at bay. (For info on the connection between inflammation and chronic illnesses, turn to Chapter 3.)

In this section, we discuss the four kinds of fats that show up on nutrition labels: saturated fats, monounsaturated fats, polyunsaturated fats, and trans fats.

It's all good: Identifying unsaturated fats

Unsaturated fats are the best fats. You find unsaturated fats largely in plant-based foods, such as olive oil, avocado oils, and cashews, as well as in fish.

Unsaturated fats may be monounsaturated or polyunsaturated. Here's how these fats differ:

✔ **Monounsaturated fats:** Monounsaturated are typically liquid at room temperature, but they solidify if chilled. These fats can help lower bad cholesterol levels and lower your risk of heart disease and stroke. Sources of monounsaturated fats also provide some nutrients that help maintain your body's cell membranes and are typically high in the anti-oxidant vitamin E.

✔ **Polyunsaturated fats:** Polyunsaturated fats are liquid at room temperature and remain in liquid form even when chilled. Polyunsaturated fats work to lower bad cholesterol levels, and they also provide some essential fatty acids your body can't produce on its own: omega-6 and omega-3. We describe these essential fatty acids in the section "Getting your fair share of essential fatty acids: Omega-3 and omega-6" later in this chapter.

Monounsaturated and polyunsaturated fats are good for you, but remember that they still contain a lot of calories. Moderation is key.

Seeing the bad in (most) saturated fats

Most saturated fats are derived from animal fats — eggs, meat, and dairy — but you can also find them in some plant sources, such as palm and coconut.

Saturated fats tend to fall on the do-not-eat list and with good reason. They're solid fats that often work to clog your arteries and raise the LDL cholesterol — the bad cholesterol. Saturated fats have also been linked to an increased risk of stroke. They concentrate fat-soluble toxins from your environment that can disrupt the cell-to-cell communication and contribute to chronic metabolic disease.

Chemistry stuff: Understanding fat names

Chemically speaking, fats are composed of hydrogen, carbon, and oxygen atoms. Fats may be named for the number of carbon atoms they have, and the number of double bonds between their carbon atoms, the locations of those double bonds, and more. All this info is important for biochemists because the shape and size of the fat molecule determines how it'll behave and react with other molecules in the body.

Whether a fat is saturated or unsaturated depends on the number of hydrogen atoms. A saturated fat contains the maximum number of hydrogen atoms. An unsaturated fat has at least one place where carbon atoms form an extra bond with each other — a *double bond* — instead of attaching to another hydrogen atom. Saturated fats have no double bonds between the carbon atoms, monounsaturated fats have one double bond between carbon atoms, and polyunsaturated fats have more than one double bond. Double bonds make the molecule more rigid and may give it a bent shape.

For unsaturated fats, names can also indicate the location of the double bond. For example, omega-3 fatty acids have their double bond three carbon atoms away from the end. Omega-6s have it six carbons away from the end.

Trans refers to the way the hydrogen atoms are arranged in 3-D space in relation to a double bond. Molecules with trans configurations tend to be locked in a fairly straight shape, so they get clogged in the arteries more easily than other fats.

Of course, some types of saturated fats are better than others. There are many different kinds of saturated fatty acids, each with a different chemical makeup. Medium- and short-chain fatty acids, like the lauric acid found in coconut oil, have been shown to be beneficial for the immune system and gastrointestinal cells. That's why coconut oil is on our anti-inflammatory food list even though it's a saturated fat.

The American Heart Association recommends staying away from saturated fats. Because saturated fat is hard to avoid altogether, the AHA suggests that the calories from saturated fats not exceed 7 percent of the total calories you take in for the day. In other words, on a 2,000-calorie diet, only 140 calories should come from saturated fat.

The worst of the bunch: Avoiding trans fats

Trans fats have no nutritional value whatsoever. Unlike the other fats, trans fats are almost entirely artificial, although they do appear in very small amounts in some meats.

Trans fats are made through a process called *hydrogenation* or *partial hydrogenation,* in which producers expose an otherwise-healthy monounsaturated fat like vegetable oil to heat and fill it with hydrogen atoms, turning it into a solid fat. It's an ideal fat for the commercial food industry because of its smooth texture and reusability in deep frying. Trans fats also extend the shelf-life of foods, making it perfect for packaged pastries.

Not only do trans fats increase the levels of LDL (bad) cholesterol, but they also counteract any HDL (good) cholesterol that may be in a particular food. Trans fats are so unhealthy, in fact, that they've been the target of health campaigns since about 2000, with many restaurants and commercial vendors promising to reduce the amount of trans fats. Some have actually succeeded: Although margarine was initially filled with trans fats in its solid form, many producers have eliminated trans fats, which makes even the sticks more spreadable.

Be on the lookout for "partially hydrogenated" oils in ingredients lists. The product contains trans fats, even if the label says the amount of trans fats per serving is 0 grams. If the total per serving is less than 0.5 grams, manufacturers are allowed to list it as 0 grams.

Identifying the Best Fat Sources

You can find fat in plenty of places, that's for sure. But to find the *good* fats, the ones that help your body do what it's supposed to do, you have to look just a little harder. Knowing how to look and what to look for can mean the difference between successfully moving on to an anti-inflammatory diet and giving up much too soon.

Table 5-1 is a useful reference for figuring out which foods supply your body with the different types of fat. Use this information to help you decide which foods to eat and which foods to avoid based on their fats. Monounsaturated and polyunsaturated fats are the good fats; saturated and trans fats are the bad fats.

Table 5-1	Sources of Good and Bad Fats		
Monounsaturated	*Polyunsaturated*	*Saturated*	*Trans*
Avocado	Salmon, mackerel, herring, trout, sardines	Fatty meats	Biscuits
Olive oil, olives	Cod liver oil	Lard	Cakes
Almonds, pecans, brazil nuts, hazelnuts, cashews, peanuts	Soybeans	Chicken skin	Pastries
Sunflower oil and seeds	Walnuts	Butter, cream, full-cream milk, cheese, ice cream	Doughnuts
Sesame oil and seeds	Flaxseed, flaxseed oil	Coconut oil (a good saturated fat)	Shortening
Grapeseed oil	Grapeseed oil	Palm oil	Many margarines
Oatmeal	Wheat germ	Deep fried foods, fast food	Microwave popcorn

You know that some dietary fat is necessary, but how much is enough? Limit total fat intake to 20 to 30 percent of your daily calories, or 40 to 60 grams of total fat a day. Here's a list of recommendations for daily fat intake according to each type:

- **Monounsaturated and polyunsaturated fats:** There are no specific recommendations for unsaturated fats, but most of your fats should be unsaturated. Concentrate on eating foods with these kinds of fats while keeping within your total fat requirements.

- **Saturated fat:** Nutritional guidelines call for no more than 20 grams of saturated fats for a 2,000 calorie diet. Less is ideal.

- **Trans fat:** Nutritionists don't give a specific number but say the less you consume, the better. The American Heart Association recommends limiting trans fats to 1 percent of your total calories or fewer, preferably less than 2 grams per day.

In this section, we discuss sources of fat in more detail.

Getting your fair share of essential fatty acids: Omega-3 and omega-6

Essential fatty acids are a necessary part of your diet, especially if you're hoping to fight inflammation. "Essential" fats are those your body can't assemble — you need to receive these fats from your diet on a regular basis. Daily fish oils or fish oil supplements can help maintain good blood levels of this anti-inflammatory fat.

Omega-3 fatty acids are a kind of *essential fatty acid* (EFA) that not only help reduce the risk of heart disease and stroke but also help diminish the symptoms of anxiety, depression, attention deficit disorder, joint pain, and even some skin problems. Omega-3 fats work because they encourage the body to create the chemicals that fight inflammation. Just as important, though, is their ability to ward off the inflammatory effects of another essential fatty acid, omega-6.

For maximal anti-inflammatory benefit, you want at least a 2:1 ratio of omega-3 versus omega-6 in your diet.

The following are excellent sources of omega-3 fatty acids:

- ✔ Nut oils, fish oils
- ✔ Salmon, mackerel, halibut, sardines
- ✔ Omega-3-enriched eggs
- ✔ Chia seeds
- ✔ Hemp
- ✔ Flaxseeds and flaxseed oil
- ✔ Pumpkin seeds
- ✔ Persian walnuts

The following are good sources of omega-6 fatty acids:

- ✔ Vegetable oils
- ✔ Walnuts, cashews, almonds, Brazil nuts
- ✔ Flaxseeds, sesame seeds, pumpkin seeds, sunflower seeds

Exploring cooking oils

Here are the benefits of some cooking oils you may want to consider on an anti-inflammatory diet:

✔ **Olive oil:** In addition to being made up of monounsaturated fats, olive oil boasts a number of other benefits. It contains iron, vitamin K, and many of the same antioxidants found in fruits and vegetables. Extra-virgin olive oil decreases inflammation, helps with insulin resistance, has antibacterial properties, and helps to retain the anti-inflammatory properties of the food that you're cooking and eating.

All olive oils have the same amount of fat, so if you don't like the lighter oil, go for some that's a bit heavier. Keep in mind, however, that non-virgin olive oil doesn't have as many antioxidant polyphenols, which may help prevent heart disease and some cancers.

✔ **Sesame oil:** Sesame oil, with all its essential fatty acid benefits, not only helps lower cholesterol but also benefits the heart and kidneys. It's high in linoleic acid — one of the necessary EFAs — which helps prevent arthritis, hair loss, mood swings, and sometimes heart, liver, and kidney disease. Unrefined sesame oil also contains antioxidants, which battle free radicals and help prevent degenerative disease.

Sesame oil is an omega-6 fatty acid, and in order to retain its healthful benefits, you should balance it with at least as much omega-3 fatty acid.

✔ **Sunflower oil:** According to the National Sunflower Association, sunflower oil, made from oil-type sunflower seeds, is a light-tasting oil that's higher in vitamin E than other vegetable oils. This characteristic is beneficial in an anti-inflammatory diet because of vitamin E's ability to help lower the risk of heart disease and cancer.

Look for high oleic sunflower oil, keeping in mind that because sunflower oil is an omega-6 fatty acid, it must be balanced with omega-3 foods and oils.

✔ **Coconut oil:** Coconut oil is the exception to the rule: Made up almost 90 percent saturated fat, it's still considered one of the healthy oils. Despite its high concentration of saturated fats, that fat is about 50 percent lauric acid, which helps in preventing heart problems. The antioxidants in coconut oil make it effective as an anti-aging oil, and it can be helpful in preventing degenerative diseases.

Coconut oil is a good substitute for butter in baking — use the same amount of coconut oil as you would butter.

Getting to the meat of the issue: Animal fats

Here's something you may not know: Animal fats are good for you, as long as they come from a healthy animal. By "healthy," we mean that the animal should have been kept from drugs, antibiotics, hormone injections, or anything else used to make the meat bigger and better. The animal should also have had an appropriate diet.

Meat from organically raised, pastured (grass-fed) animals has the nutrients you need without the harmful chemicals. Meat and other products from grain-fed animals have about a 15:1 ratio of omega-6 to omega-3 fats, whereas grass-fed meat has a less inflammatory ratio at 1:1.

The problem is that grain tends to be the cheapest thing to feed the animals due to government subsidies, and the majority of meat on the market today comes from animals that have been shot up with antibiotics and growth hormones to bulk them up.

Finding organically grown, pasture-raised meat is getting easier. Many grocery stores keep a bit of a supply on hand, and farmer's markets can also be good sources of quality meats. Here's a website for a market that can deliver the meat to your door: www.grasslandbeef.com. The prices for organic, pasture-raised meat are higher, but the supply should increase as producers notice the demand, bringing prices down.

Dairy products are also a good source of animal fat for people who can tolerate lactose, but it's best in lowfat varieties and in moderation. Dairy products made from sheep's milk or goat's milk are healthier alternatives that are often more easily tolerated than cow's milk. As with meat, opt for milk from organically raised, grass-fed animals.

Finding other good fats in your diet

Here are some healthy places to find good fats:

- ✓ **Coconut fat:** Although coconut fat is a little more than 90 percent saturated fat, it's considered a healthy fat. More than 60 percent of coconut fat is made up of medium-chain triglycerides (MCTs), and half of that consists of a strong antimicrobial fatty acid called lauric acid. Lauric acid helps build up a healthy immune system.

- ✓ **Dark chocolate:** Look for chocolate that's more than 70 percent cocoa. Cocoa is very rich in antioxidants and monounsaturated fatty acids. Try to keep the treat down to just one or two small pieces.

By now you should be thinking to yourself, "How do I get started?" That's an easy one — you just decide to start and do it. Chapter 16 tells you how to turn your kitchen into a healthy food haven just by tossing a few things out and replacing them with healthier options.

Chapter 6

Conquering Carbohydrates

*T*hink of your body as your house. To make everything in your house work, you need energy. It keeps the lights on, powers the computer and television, and keeps the refrigerator running. You can use many different kinds of energy sources for your house — electric, gas, solar, and so on. Some kinds are environmentally friendly, and others may require additional resources to be fueled and therefore run just a bit slower.

Similarly, your body needs energy to do all the things it needs to do, from standing and thinking to running a marathon. It even needs energy to sleep (a lot goes on in your body while you're sleeping!). That's where carbohydrates come in. Carbohydrates are your body's source of quick energy. Compared to fats and proteins, little is needed for the body to break down carbs and release their energy. Carbs keep you moving, inside and out.

Like those energy sources for your house, however, some energy sources are better than others. Good carbohydrate sources can make your body run efficiently, but others make you feel sluggish. The key is knowing the difference and regulating your diet so that you get the right carbs in the right amounts to help fight inflammation.

This chapter takes a closer look at types of carbohydrates. We also cover carbohydrate sources — grains, fruits and vegetables, and some refined foods — and why you need to be aware of the role each plays in an anti-inflammatory diet. A common source of carbohydrates is wheat products, which create inflammation in people with allergies, sensitivities, or intolerances to wheat or gluten. Fortunately, there are many other healthy gluten-free sources of carbohydrates, and we discuss them here.

Understanding the Role of Carbohydrates

Here are the main functions of carbohydrates:

- ✔ Providing energy for the muscles and central nervous system
- ✔ Preventing protein from being used as energy
- ✔ Enabling fatty acid breakdown for fats and energy
- ✔ Providing the body with sources of fiber to keep the digestive system healthy

Sugars are the building blocks of carbohydrates. After you eat something that contains carbohydrates — usually something from the grains, fruits, vegetables, and dairy groups — the carb is broken down into simple sugars, such as glucose and fructose.

Carbohydrate digestion begins in the mouth with enzymes in the saliva breaking down starch into simpler carbohydrates. The stomach isn't involved in the breakdown of carbohydrates; that occurs in the small intestine with enzymes from the pancreas and brush border enzymes from the small intestine. After carbohydrates from a meal are broken down into simple sugars, they can be absorbed into the bloodstream. Body cells can pull in the glucose and directly use it for energy, and simple sugars such as fructose go to the liver for processing.

At this point, things may get a little hectic: If the body doesn't need glucose for energy, it stores it as *glycogen* in the liver and muscles. Glycogen is kind of the backup system to the glucose — your body uses it when the glucose supplies are too low for the activity needing energy. But if the storage units for glycogen are full, the glucose gets stored as fat.

Glucose is the primary source of energy for all the body's cells. The body also uses fats and protein for energy but only indirectly — after your body has first converted them into glucose. By using carbohydrates for energy, the body can save protein for its intended use: as a building block for muscle and tissue development and maintenance.

Carbohydrates give your body and brain quick energy, but that energy can't be sustained without proteins and fats.

Types of Carbs: Comparing Simple and Complex Carbohydrates

Just as there are good and bad fats, there are good and bad carbohydrates. Carbohydrates may be simple or complex. Simple carbohydrates, or *simple sugars,* have just one or two sugar units *(saccharides). Complex carbohydrates,* also known as *starches* or *polysaccharides,* typically have chains of three or more linked sugars. You can find them in foods such as grain, bread, oatmeal, rice, and even vegetables like broccoli and corn.

Both simple and complex carbohydrates go through the process of being broken down and converted into glucose, the leftover of which is then converted into glycogen — all of which is done through a process called *glucose metabolism.* Here's how simple and complex carbs differ:

- ✔ **Simple carbohydrates:** The simple carbohydrates — made of only one or two sugar units — are broken into sugar almost immediately when digested and go straight for the bloodstream. The simple carbohydrates in processed or refined foods, such as candy bars, are the most inflammatory and are considered empty calories. These foods have been stripped of healthful nutrients and buffers for blood-sugar regulation. We specifically discuss sugar and other sweeteners in Chapter 8.

  Although many simple-carbohydrate sources are considered bad, fruits and many vegetables contain simple sugars such as fructose. However, other nutrients and fiber make the advantages of these simple-carb sources far outweigh the costs.

- ✔ **Complex carbohydrates:** These carbohydrates — made of three or more sugar units — usually take longer to go through glucose metabolism because the body has to do more work to take them apart.

Imagine you're running a marathon. You have a long distance ahead of you. Are you going to spread your energy out over time, or are you going to push hard in the beginning, only to wear out before you hit the halfway mark? Your body is doing that marathon, and it's counting on you to make the right choices. Simple carbohydrates give you a quick boost, but when that boost is over, you may feel even more tired, rundown, and sluggish than before.

Fiber is a carbohydrate that's so complex that the body can't break it down for energy, so it passes through the body undigested. Although fiber isn't an energy source, it helps keep your bowels healthy, lowers blood cholesterol, and helps control blood sugar levels. See the later section "Going complex and unrefined" later in this chapter for details.

Keeping Carbs in Check to Help Inflammation

High blood sugar is one of the top causes of inflammation, and one of the main nutrients leading to elevated blood sugar is carbohydrates. It makes sense, then, that if you're struggling with inflammation you should cut out your carbs, right?

Not so fast. Focusing on carbohydrates can help reduce the risk of inflammation, but that doesn't mean cutting them out completely; it just means reining them in. One strong step in lowering your inflammation is lowering the amount of carbohydrates you take in, making sure that what carbs you *do* have are the complex carbs. In this section, we discuss simple and refined carbohydrates, the glycemic index, complex carbohydrates, and the amounts of carbs you need.

The not-so-simple truth about simple carbs

Simple carbohydrates, or simple sugars, tend to be the dangerous ones — the ones that are secretly tucked away in your top drawer at work or behind your favorite sweater in the closet at home. They're the ones you know you shouldn't eat, the ones made with refined sugars that are broken down quickly but come with very few useful vitamins or minerals. The worst sources of simple carbohydrates are foods made with refined sugars and/or refined flours, dietary no-nos we cover in Chapter 2.

Most of the foods you find on any naughty list are sources of simple carbohydrates: doughnuts, cakes, pastries, candy bars, soda, white breads. They're not as good for you as complex carbohydrates because the body breaks them into simple sugars so quickly.

Fruits contain the simple sugar *fructose,* but fruit is rarely a problem in moderation because of the other nutrients and fiber it contains. The overall sugar content in each serving of fruit is low. However, when fructose is concentrated and you eat a lot of it — as in table sugar and high-fructose corn syrup, which are both half fructose — the impact on the body can be very different. Fructose is processed by the liver, and in high amounts, fructose contributes to insulin resistance and inflammation.

Bewaring refined carbs

You're walking through an orchard, and all of a sudden you see it: the most beautiful, ripest, reddest apple you've ever seen. You pick it, rub it on your shirt to get a nice shine . . . and just before you take a bite, someone stops you. Before you can eat that apple, it must be sprayed, peeled, cored, diced and put into a pot. A syrup made up of sugar and a list of ingredients you can't pronounce is poured over the top. It's all stirred together, poured into a bowl and handed back to you. It just doesn't seem the same, does it?

That's what happens when foods are refined. Whole foods — grains, sugars, fruits, vegetables — are taken apart and processed. In many cases, the healthy parts of the original food are stripped out, the food is bleached, and in the end, the food looks nothing like it did in the beginning. Throughout the process, the food lost vitamins, nutrients, and everything else that made it a wholesome food in the first place.

When the food loses its vitamins and other nutrients, it also loses its ability to fight inflammation. In most cases, refined and processed foods become inflammatory, furthering any damage that may exist.

Refined sugars and flours have been stripped of all their nutrients; put them together, throw in a few chemical preservatives, and you have an inflammatory nightmare. Because of this process, the body digests these carbs rapidly, leading to a spike in blood sugar and later ending with a crash.

If you're eating a diet high in processed foods, the following things may happen to your body as a result:

- ✔ **Rapidly changing blood sugar:** Processed foods tend to be high in sugar, and the sugar goes into your bloodstream faster and at a higher volume than your body can handle. The rapid increase in blood sugar kicks your pancreas into overdrive in creating insulin. The insulin (if it works properly) lowers the blood sugar, but often at a pace faster than your body can handle. Otherwise, the blood sugar remains elevated.

- ✔ **Cavities:** Cavities may seem like a minor problem by comparison, but unhealthy teeth and gums can affect your overall health. Refined sugars are in all regular soft drinks, which enter the mouth in high concentrations.

- ✔ **Increased appetite and weight gain:** The National Institutes for Health considers refined carbohydrates to be *empty calories*. That means basically their only nutritional value is a caloric one, which isn't much of a value at all to your health. In fact, often the sugars in those foods trick your body into thinking it's hungry when it's not — which in turn makes you think you need to eat. This cycle not only hinders weight loss but also contributes to weight gain.

  Refined carbohydrates also raise blood sugar levels too quickly, causing the body to increase insulin production, which then promotes fat production and fat storage.

The problem is that refined carbohydrates are everywhere, often hiding in places you wouldn't expect to find them. Sweetened fruit juices, often made with high-fructose corn syrup, have refined carbohydrates, as do some frozen or canned fruits and vegetables. Reduced-fat snacks often contain extra sugar to make up for the changes in flavor and texture that occurred when the fat was cut. White rice and pasta are great places to find refined carbs as well.

Watching for the sugar rush: The glycemic index and glycemic load

Simple versus complex isn't the whole story in carbs. After all, some carbohydrates are more complex than others. For example, starchy white potatoes don't pose much of a challenge to the carb-breaking enzymes of your digestive system. Your body quickly breaks the starch into the simple sugar glucose, which then enters your bloodstream.

Other factors besides a carb's complexity influence a food's effect on blood sugar. For example, fats, protein, and fiber can slow digestion or limit absorption of glucose, and even the makeup of the carb can affect how much blood sugar fluctuates. You sometimes get glucose simply by breaking the carb apart in the intestines; at other times, simple sugars have to go to the liver for processing.

The *glycemic index* (GI) is a numerical rating based on a food's *glycemic response,* or how quickly the body converts it into glucose. The index uses a scale of 0 to 100, with the higher scores going to those foods that cause the most rapid rise in blood sugar. You can look up GI values at www.glycemic index.com.

When gauging the effect on blood sugar, you also need to consider the amount of carbs you eat. The *glycemic load* (GL) is the formula describing the body's glycemic response based on both the type of carbohydrate and the amount you consume. Peanuts, for example, have a glycemic index of 14, but eating just 4 ounces — which comes to about 15 net carbs — yields a glycemic load of just 2.

The mathematical formula for the glycemic load is fairly simple:

$$GL = (GI/100) \times \text{Net Carbs}$$

where Net Carbs are total carbohydrates per serving minus dietary fiber.

Going complex and unrefined

Keeping the good carbs — the unrefined and complex carbohydrates — a regular part of your diet can help fight inflammation and chronic illness. If you have diabetes or blood sugar issues, make sure you also look at the glycemic load (GL) of carbohydrate-rich foods (we discuss the GL in the preceding section). Even whole foods containing complex carbohydrates raise blood sugar.

A diet filled with complex carbohydrates coupled with dark, leafy vegetables such as spinach is one of the best ways to fight inflammation naturally. The leafy vegetables are a good source of phytochemicals and antioxidants, both of which fight inflammation. Good sources of complex carbohydrates include blueberries, beans, barley, buckwheat, lentils, whole-grain cereals, chickpeas, broccoli, spinach, and oats.

Fiber is another good carbohydrate that can help fight inflammation. There are two kinds of fiber:

- **Soluble fiber:** Soluble fiber helps control blood sugar and may also help lower cholesterol. Sources of soluble fiber include oat bran, natural oatmeal, beans, sweet potatoes, carrots, peas, strawberries, bananas, rice bran, barley, and citrus.

- **Insoluble fiber:** This carb may be beneficial in helping to lower the risk of colon cancer and keeping the bowel functioning the way it should. Some healthy sources of insoluble fiber include cabbage, beets, Brussels sprouts, turnips, cauliflower, barley, and whole-wheat breads, bran, and cereals.

Nutrients such as vitamin C make a carb source — even a simple-sugar source such as fruit — have health benefits in helping the body to do things like scavenge free-radical damage. Unrefined and complex carbohydrate sources contain the vitamins, minerals, fiber, and other nutrients you need for your brain and body to function at its best and continue to fight inflammation.

Calculating your carb needs

On an anti-inflammatory diet, fill up at least half (50 to 75 percent) of your plate with complex carbohydrates in the form of vegetables, whole grains, legumes, and low-glycemic-index fruit. When you add in vegetable protein sources (see Chapter 7) that contain complex carbohydrates, three-fourths of your plate will be taken by these foods.

Here's a simple clue: Each gram of carbohydrates provides 4 calories. So first figure what 60 percent of your daily caloric goal is: If you're on a 2,000 calorie diet, multiply 2,000 by 60 percent: 1,200 calories should come from carbohydrates. Then take that number and divide by 4 — the number of calories per gram of carbohydrate; 1,200 calories divided by 4 calories per gram is 300 grams of carbohydrates each day.

You should have three to five servings of complex carbohydrates each day — but that doesn't mean you should have five servings of pizza or five big bowls of breakfast cereal. You can easily put together a daily menu that includes yogurt (if you can tolerate dairy), brown rice, broccoli, yams, and an apple for a treat. Keeping the foods to an anti-inflammatory list narrows the menu selection a bit — for example, you may have pizza made on whole-grain wheat-free flatbread with goat cheese — but it's far from impossible.

Need a visual? Divide your plate into four sections. Leave two sections for vegetable-related carbohydrates and one for whole grains. The remaining section is for your protein.

Choosing Your Carb Sources

Nutritionally speaking, carbohydrates should make up about 40 percent of your daily caloric intake. That sounds like a lot of carbs, especially when you've been saturated with news about how bad carbs are for you. But sticking to good carbohydrates — the complex, unrefined carbohydrates — over the bad ones can ward off inflammation and help you feel better inside and out.

The closer a food looks to its natural state, the better it is for you. Fresh fruits and vegetables are usually a good pick when looking for a healthy food with good carbohydrates. An added bonus: Stocking up on fresh fruits and vegetables means not having to study nutrition labels!

Other natural carb sources include whole grains, barley, and brown rice — the grains as they would appear before they're stripped of their nutrients and refined. Choose brown rice over white, whole-grain pasta over enriched, and natural oats over the packets with the flavoring and sugar.

In this section, we help you select your grains and fruits and vegetables, and we explain how to interpret the carb content of packaged foods.

Adding great grains to your diet

They don't call grains the "staff of life" without reason. Grains have a significant historical value to the legacy of human survival and continue to be an essential part of a healthy diet. *Grains* are the seeds of different types of grasses, and they come in various sizes, shapes, and textures.

For most people, grains are a major source of complex carbohydrates as well as several vitamins and minerals. The grains that haven't been refined — whole grains — take that health benefit a few steps further.

Enjoying yourself with whole grains

A diet rich in whole grains can be a very full diet indeed, as well as one that doesn't leave you feeling like you're missing out. Whole grains have a plethora of health benefits — not the least of which is the reduced risk of several chronic diseases — and this kind of diet is just plain *good*.

Aside from tasting good, whole grains really are good for you. The fiber in whole grains helps reduce the risk of coronary heart disease and may help with weight management and bowel function. For women who are pregnant, eating folate-fortified grains helps prevent some defects that may occur during fetal development.

Here are some additional diverse benefits of whole grains:

✔ Grains are an important source of several B vitamins, such as thiamin, riboflavin, folate, and niacin, and of minerals, such as iron and magnesium, all of which aid the body in releasing energy from proteins, fats, and carbohydrates.

✔ The magnesium in whole grains helps build bones, and the selenium helps protect cells from oxidation. Oxidation is what happens when reactive oxygen molecules called *free radicals* attack your body.

✔ Dietary fiber from whole grains can help lower the risk of heart disease and lower cholesterol.

✔ Whole grains are a great source of iron, especially for people who don't eat red meat.

A sensitive topic: Getting complex carbs with gluten-free grains

Not everyone's body can tolerate whole grains that contain the protein gluten. In fact, for people with celiac disease, even the smallest amount of gluten can damage the small intestine and prevent it from absorbing nutrients (see Chapter 2). Gluten proteins are in all forms of wheat — including durum, semolina, spelt, kamut, einkorn, and faro — and in related grains, such as rye, barley, and triticale.

All is not lost, however. The Celiac Sprue Association, the largest nonprofit celiac support group in the United States, provides a Grains and Flours Glossary on its website (www.csaceliacs.org/gluten_grains.php) so people avoiding gluten can get all the benefits of their wheat-eating counterparts. Some of the gluten-free substitutions they suggest include the following:

- **Acorn:** It's a sweet, edible nut that you can use whole or ground into flour. The flour adds flavor and fiber but doesn't bind well when baking.

- **Almond:** Almond is another sweet, edible nut that can be used whole or ground into flour. You can use almond flour alone or with other flours in cakes, pastries, and breads.

- **Amaranth:** Amaranth is a tiny seed related to spinach and beets. Seeds are available whole or ground into a light-brown flour. Amaranth is vitamin-rich, provides several minerals, and contains about 30 percent more protein than wheat flour, rice, and oats.

- **Beans:** Beans are the seeds of plants in the legume family. You can use them whole as a cooked vegetable, pureed as a thickener, or dried and ground into flour. Many gluten-free bean flours are available commercially.

- **Brown rice:** Brown rice is made of rice kernels from which only the hull has been removed. Cooked brown rice has a slightly chewy texture and a nut-like flavor.

Stocking up on the right fruits and veggies

Complex carbohydrates are mainly fibers and starches, which you find in plant foods such as vegetables. Simple carbohydrates include the sugars from fruits. So does that mean fruits, which are chock full of vitamins, minerals, and other nutrients, have to fall off your menu? Not at all.

Not only do fruits have a lot of the same carbohydrates as other foods, but they also give you the additional benefits of vitamins, minerals, fiber, and phytochemicals, those plant compounds that have antioxidant and anti-inflammatory benefits. An apple, for example, has about 44 calories and 10 grams of carbohydrates, whereas a serving of potato chips has 150 calories and 15 grams of carbs. Choose the chips, and you get more calories, more carbs — and not the good kind — and far fewer vitamins, fiber, antioxidants, and minerals.

As for vegetables, you can hardly go wrong. That's not to say you can't go wrong, just that it's harder to do so. Your best bet for good carbohydrate value is to turn to reds, oranges, and dark greens, such as beets, sweet potatoes, and spinach. Iceberg lettuce, on the other hand, has little to no nutritional value.

The more colors in your fruit and vegetable rainbow, the better. The colors come from antioxidant-rich compounds, such as *carotenoids,* the cancer-fighting orange pigment found in carrots.

Making your produce picks

In this section we list just a few of the fruits and vegetables that contribute to a healthy level of carbohydrates and at the same time help fight inflammation and chronic illness. Here are some good fruit choices for carbohydrates:

- ✔ **Apricots:** 4 grams per whole apricot
- ✔ **Blueberries:** 14.5 grams per cup
- ✔ **Cantaloupe:** 6 grams per wedge
- ✔ **Cherries:** 16 grams per cup
- ✔ **Grapefruit:** 23 grams per whole grapefruit
- ✔ **Honeydew:** 9 grams per wedge
- ✔ **Kiwi:** 14.66 grams per cup
- ✔ **Orange:** 16 grams per orange
- ✔ **Peaches:** 15 grams per whole medium peach
- ✔ **Pears:** 15.46 grams per pear
- ✔ **Raspberries:** 15 grams per cup
- ✔ **Tangerines:** 12 grams per whole medium tangerine

And here are some vegetable choices and their carb contents:

- ✔ **Dark leafy greens:** 1.6 grams per serving
- ✔ **Hearty greens (kale, collard):** 3.7 grams per serving
- ✔ **Carrot:** 7 grams per carrot
- ✔ **Bok choy:** 1.5 grams per serving
- ✔ **Cabbage:** 1.9 grams per serving
- ✔ **Celery:** 1.5 grams per stalk
- ✔ **Radishes:** 1 gram each
- ✔ **Mushrooms:** 1.4 grams per serving
- ✔ **Okra:** 7.5 grams per cup

When buying produce, fresh is best. But when fresh isn't possible, choose frozen. Be sure to check the labels to see how the food was frozen and whether it contains chemicals or other preservatives. Although whole fruits and vegetables are great choices, often the fruit juices or fruit juice concentrates have too much concentrated fructose — the natural sugars in fruit — or added sugars and can be considered a bad carbohydrate.

Eating locally and in season

Eating fresh fruits and vegetables is good for you in so many ways, and it's even better when you're eating it at the right time. Pick something off the vine too soon, and you don't get the taste or texture — and certainly not the nutrients — you were expecting. Eating local fruits and vegetables in season also allows you to get the highest nutrient content because the food doesn't have to be shipped long distances or stored long-term. The food can be picked ripe, often within days or hours of your eating it.

Here's a short list of when various fruits and vegetables come in season:

- ✔ **Citrus:** Winter and spring
- ✔ **Greens (lettuce, spinach, arugula, and so on):** Most are good year-round but best in spring
- ✔ **Berries:** Mid to late summer
- ✔ **Melons:** Summer and early fall
- ✔ **Root vegetables:** Can be planted over and over and have healthy harvests spring through fall

For more-detailed info on when local produce is in season, search online for a harvest calendar specific to your state.

Opting for organics

Chances are you're considering an anti-inflammation diet because you want to feel better, be healthier, and avoid as many chronic illnesses as possible. If you're going to take the time to rework your menu to include fresh fruits and vegetables, why not go a step further and try to eat mostly organic?

There are definite advantages to buying organically grown fruits and vegetables, especially if you're lucky enough to live near a farmer's market or an organic market where the produce sold is locally grown. When that happens, you know — or have a good idea — who grew the food and what kind of soil it grew in.

Organic fruits and vegetables are grown without pesticides or herbicides. They're not injected with anything to boost their color, and they're not genetically modified to become some kind of food-seller's super food — one that survives long shipping, is more resistant to colder weather, or is bigger than normal (often at the expense of flavor and texture).

If you can't buy all your fruits and vegetables organic, be selective. An organization called the Environmental Working Group (EWG) put together a list called the "Dirty Dozen" that includes the 12 fruits and vegetables that you should buy organic due to commercial pesticide contamination. Here are those fruits and vegetables, starting with the most contaminated:

- ✔ Celery

- ✔ Peaches

- ✔ Strawberries

- ✔ Apples

- ✔ Blueberries

- ✔ Nectarines

- ✔ Sweet bell peppers

- ✔ Spinach

- ✔ Cherries

- ✔ Kale/collard greens

- ✔ Potatoes

- ✔ Imported grapes

Onions, avocados, and pineapples top the clean list.

According to the EWG, eating the 12 most contaminated fruits and vegetables exposes a person to an average of 15 pesticides a day. Eating from the clean list exposes a person to about 2 pesticides. You can catch the full list in EWG's Shopper's Guide to Pesticides (www.foodnews.org).

Checking the labels on packaged foods

What about the things you should stay away from? Creating a healthy life-style means making changes — both additions and deletions. Some foods are good in moderation, but some things — refined or processed foods — you should avoid whenever possible. But for those times when you do eat pack-aged foods, you should know how to interpret a food label.

When it comes to carbohydrates, know that carbs can be divided into three main parts: fiber, sugars, and starches. (You should also know, however, that there are some parts of carbohydrates that aren't required to be listed on the nutrition label.) The food label will typically give you the amount of carbs in a serving size and list what percentage of your daily allowance of carbs that serving provides. Directly under the carbs heading will be the particles of the carbs broken down: a ½-cup serving of frozen Brussels sprouts, for instance, has 6 grams total carbs, with 2 grams each of sugars and fiber. The remain-ing 2 grams isn't listed on the label and is likely made up of those "phantom" parts.

Figuring out which foods are high in simple carbohydrates can be challenging; the United States Department of Agriculture (USDA) recommends that when checking food labels, you keep an eye out for certain clue words: fructose, dextrose, sucrose, malt sugar, and high-fructose corn syrup. They may be hiding in an otherwise healthy food.

Chapter 7

Getting the Right Kinds of Protein

- -

In This Chapter

▶ Seeing how the body uses protein

▶ Getting to the meat of the protein issue

▶ Balancing your protein sources

- -

Ask for advice about protein, and you're bound to get a wide variety of statements: You need it. The more you exercise, the more you should have. You can't get enough without meat. You get too much if you eat meat.

The word *protein* is Greek for "of first importance," and dietary protein is vital to your survival. *Amino acids* are the building blocks of proteins. Unfortunately, humans don't have the ability to make all 22 amino acids required to make the proteins their bodies need. Your body can only make 13 of those amino acids, and the rest have to come from your diet.

Knowing which protein sources provide the best anti-inflammatory benefits without inflammatory side effects is the key to making it all work. In this chapter, we discuss protein's role in the body, its connection to inflammation, and how to balance your protein sources in your diet.

Looking at Protein's Role in the Body

Protein is an essential part of any diet, whether you're omnivore, vegetarian, vegan, or just a regular Joe who eats what he wants to eat. Your body uses protein to repair damaged tissues, build muscle, and feed your blood. Hair and nails are made up of protein, as are cartilage and bone. Hormones such as insulin are proteins, and the neurotransmitters that send messages in the brain come from amino acids, which come from dietary proteins.

Proteins are involved in a lot of cell processes. Proteins may act as *enzymes,* which cause or increase the rates of chemical reactions in the body. Proteins also determine which large molecules can pass through a membrane — the proteins ferry certain molecules across to the other side.

Proteins are important to the immune system as well. Antibodies, for example, are proteins. *C-reactive protein* (CRP) is an *acute phase protein* — one that increases or decreases in response to inflammation — made in the liver. When the body is under attack from illness or injury, the liver produces more CRP. Heightened CRP levels are a warning signal that your body is working to fight off inflammation. Over the past several decades, researchers have discovered increased CRP levels in patients suffering from heart disease, diabetes, cancer, allergies, and arthritis, including rheumatoid arthritis.

Considering Your Protein Sources

There's a common misconception that only people who follow certain dietary guidelines get the right amount of protein. In fact, you can get the "right amount" of protein, regardless of whether you're a vegetarian or you want to keep a little meat in your diet.

Just as important as finding the right amount of protein is finding the right balance of protein sources. You could get all your required protein in an all-meat diet, but two things would happen: You'd take in excessive fats, and you'd miss out on the nutrient-enriched proteins that come with plant sources. That's why meat-eaters should embrace being omnivores, eating both plant- and animal-based proteins.

In this section, we look at food sources of protein and why each one is an important part of any anti-inflammation diet.

A meat-eater's menu: Including animal sources

Mention "protein," and meat-eaters instantly think, well, meat — and it's no wonder: From a nutritional standpoint, eating both plant and animal protein sources offers health benefits over a strictly plant diet.

One of the first benefits of animal protein is the amount of amino acids it contains. Your body can't produce all the amino acids you need and must get most of them from your diet, and animal protein contains all of them. With plant sources, you usually have to mix and match to get a complete protein.

Almost all animal products contain some, and sometimes even high, amounts of protein. For example, the protein content by weight of cooked meat and poultry is between 15 and 40 percent. The bad news is those sources sometimes contain high amounts of fat. To create a good balance, you want to limit how many protein sources get more than 30 percent of their calories from fat.

Meats from grass-fed animals rather than grain-fed animals naturally have less saturated fat simply because of the animal's diet. You can also reduce unnecessary fats by choosing lean cuts and lowfat dairy products from animals that are grass-fed.

Table 7-1 lays out some animal protein sources, with their grams of protein per serving and how the fat percentage stacks up to the daily recommended allowance. *Note:* Dairy is not recommended for everyone.

Table 7-1	Animal Protein Sources	
Protein Source	*Protein*	*Fat (Percent of Daily Recommended Allowance)*
Skinless white meat chicken, roasted, 3 ounces	31 grams	26%
Skinless turkey breast, roasted, 3 ounces	24 grams	6%
Lowfat plain yogurt, 1 cup	13 grams	6%
Part skim ricotta cheese, ½ cup	10 grams	53%
Skim milk, 1 cup	8 grams	5%
One medium egg	6 grams	68%
2% milk cottage cheese, ½ cup	7 grams	17%
Cheddar cheese, 1 ounce	7 grams	70%

Taking it to the sea: Fish and seafood

You've likely heard the many benefits fish and seafood have to offer, but what exactly are they, and why do they matter? In terms of protein, fish and seafood matter quite a bit. Like their land-animal counterparts, fish and seafood provide high-quality protein in relatively high numbers.

Unlike a nice juicy burger or a thick steak, the protein you get from seafood isn't accompanied by the high levels of saturated fat and cholesterol. With the right types of seafood, you get the anti-inflammatory omega-3 fatty acids as well as vitamins and minerals. In fact, nutritionists often point to fish two to three times a week as part of a heart healthy diet.

Fish and seafood, like meat, provide all the amino acids humans can't produce. In addition to all the wonderful benefits from the omega-3 fatty acids that come from fish and seafood (see Chapter 5), 1 ounce of virtually any seafood has about 6 grams of protein. Table 7-2 lists some fish and seafood protein sources, with their grams of protein and fat percentage according to the recommended daily limits.

Table 7-2	Fish and Seafood Protein Sources	
Protein Source	*Protein*	*Fat (Percent of Daily Recommended Allowance)*
Atlantic cod, 1 4-ounce fillet	41 grams	5%
Wild salmon, 8 ounces	39 grams	20%
Sardines, canned, drained, 1 cup	37 grams	26%
Rainbow trout, 1 4-ounce fillet	33 grams	9%
Tuna, canned, in water 3 ounces	33 grams	12%
Scallops, 4 ounces	24 grams	0%
Tilapia, 3 ounces	21 grams	3%
Squid, 3 ounces	13 grams	2%
Shrimp, 4 large	5 grams	0%

Trying the vegetarian variety

One of the most common comments people who decide to go vegetarian get is "Where will you get your protein?" Most people think that without a steady diet of meat or seafood, people are protein deficient. In fact, the vegetable sources can be packed with just as much protein as their meatier counterparts but without the unnecessary fats. What's more, vegetable proteins aren't just for vegetarians — they're a great source of proteins and other nutrients for everyone.

Protein is one of the easiest nutrients to find, as long as you know what you're looking for. Here are some plant-based protein sources:

✔ **Quinoa:** Grains are a great source of protein, but the leader of the pack is quinoa. Your body needs 22 amino acids to make its proteins, and unlike most other plant-based protein sources, quinoa has them all. One cup of cooked quinoa has 18 grams of protein. What's more, quinoa is a gluten-free grain, making it safe for people with gluten sensitivities or celiac disease (see Chapter 3 for info on these conditions).

✔ **Nuts and seeds:** The best kinds of nuts and seeds — as well as the butters made from them — are almonds, cashews, and sunflower seeds. Just 2 tablespoons of almond butter (about the amount in a sandwich) has 4 grams of protein. Nuts are high in fat, but don't let that scare you — it's mostly the good fats (see Chapter 5 for info on fats).

A huge benefit of nuts and seeds is convenience. Need a little protein fix? Stop at the closest grocery or convenience store and pick up a small bag of raw nuts, such as raw almonds or cashews. Beware of nuts roasted in oil or made with sugar or honey.

✔ **Meat substitutes:** Take a look at the label of any veggie burger or seitan (a gluten meat-like product), and you may be surprised at the amount of protein. Veggie burgers contain about 10 grams of protein each, and 100 grams of seitan has about 21 grams of protein. Many Asian restaurants use seitan as a meat substitute in vegetarian dishes. (***Note:*** People with gluten sensitivities should be aware that seitan is *not* a gluten-free product.)

As with any processed food, look at the labels of meat substitutes carefully — *vegetarian* doesn't necessarily mean *healthy*. Choose meat substitutes made from beans, nuts, mushrooms, or seeds.

✔ **Soy products:** You can choose from many different ways of eating soy products and a variety of sources. Tofu, tempeh, edamame, and miso are the most popular. One of the best things about tofu is that you can determine how it's going to taste. Tofu, when blended with veggies and sauce, takes on the flavor of whatever it's cooked with. Add a little curry, and your tofu carries a bit of a kick. Another good thing about tofu? It's packed with protein: A half-cup serving has about 10 grams of protein.

Specially fermented soy products like tempeh are easier to digest than other forms.

✔ **Beans and legumes:** One powerful source of vegetable protein is the bean and legume group of foods. Often called "nature's perfect food," beans come in a wide variety of types, tastes, and textures.

Beans and legumes are inexpensive, and paired with grains such as brown rice, quinoa, or millet, they can make a hearty meal filled with all the essential amino acids you need.

Think beans are high in fat? You'd be surprised. Many varieties have less than 1 percent fat per serving — and that's the good kind of fat. Table 7-3 contains some of the most common beans and legumes (including soybean products) with their grams of protein and fat percentages.

Table 7-3	Beans and Legumes	
Protein Source	*Protein*	*Fat (Percent of Daily Recommended Allowance)*
Edamame, dry-roasted, 1 cup	68 grams	20%
Miso, 1 cup	32.1 grams	6%
Lupini beans, boiled, 1 cup	25.8 grams	3%
Lentils, boiled, 1 cup	17.9 grams	0.4%
White beans, boiled, 1 cup	17.4 grams	0.4%
Roman beans, boiled, 1 cup	16.5 grams	0.5%
Yellow beans, boiled, 1 cup	16.2 grams	1%
Kidney beans, boiled, 1 cup	15.3 grams	0.5%
Black beans, boiled, 1 cup	15.2 grams	0.5%
Great Northern beans, boiled, 1 cup	14.7 grams	0.5%

Getting the Balance Right

Protein is a vital nutrient for everyone, but people who lead more active lifestyles need slightly more protein to keep up. People with inflammation should make sure they get their daily recommended amounts of protein as an important means of keeping those issues such as obesity, cardiovascular disease, and diabetes at bay.

Fad diets have led — or *mis*led — many people to think they can eat as much protein as they like without feeling any ill effects. However, too much protein can be bad for you.

High protein/low carbohydrate diets work for weight loss because a process called *ketosis* makes the body burn its own fat rather than carbs for fuel while suppressing the appetite. The body also increases the excretion of fluids, mostly through urine, resulting in a corresponding loss of water weight. The bad news with these diets is that they provide short-term benefits like weight loss with the potential for long-term health problems. As the body breaks down the protein, higher levels of ammonia are released into the body. Also, the increased discharge of fluids means a loss of calcium, which can lead to bone and joint deterioration, even osteoporosis. Ketosis can also damage your organs, especially your liver and kidneys.

The body can't store protein after breaking it down, so your body does need to replenish its supply daily. How much protein a body needs depends on the size of that body.

The Food and Nutrition Board of the National Academy of Sciences created a Recommended Daily Allowance (RDA) cheat sheet for a variety of nutrients based on a person's age and weight. The RDA for adults is about 0.36 grams of protein for every pound of weight. If you weigh 120 pounds, you should have about 43 grams of protein a day. At 180 pounds, that increases to 65 grams of protein.

Just as important as the right amount of protein is making sure you're getting the right kinds of protein from all sources. You should have meat only two to four times a week and seafood just three times weekly (see Chapter 4 for details). The rest of your protein should come from plant-based sources. If you're eating meat for every meal, you've run up your limit by the end of Day 2.

Vegetarians must take care to eat a variety of plant-based protein sources — including beans, legumes, and grains — to get all the essential amino acids.

Chapter 8

Indulging in Sweets

In This Chapter

▶ Avoiding refined sugars and artificial sweeteners

▶ Identifying the sweets and treats that are okay in moderation

Sweetened coffee and tea, sweet rolls, pastries, ice cream — many people just can't get enough. In fact, most Americans consume more than 160 pounds of sugar each year! When changing to a diet designed to lower inflammation, however, *sweet* can be a four-letter word.

Refined sugars and foods with high sugar levels suppress your immune system and raise insulin levels, opening the door for inflammation (see Chapter 2). When blood sugar rises too rapidly, biochemical changes in the body's cells start taking place, leading to inflammation-related problems such as diabetes and heart disease, among others.

That's not to say no sweets are allowed ever again, but it's a good idea to keep processed sweets at a minimum and to replace refined sugars, refined carbohydrates, and artificial sweeteners with the natural sweeteners your body can process without leading to inflammation. In this chapter, we discuss types of sweeteners and suggest ways to safely satisfy your sweet tooth.

Connecting Sugars and Sweeteners to Inflammation

Virtually all foods made from refined sugars and artificial sweeteners — and even some natural sweeteners — have a hand in causing inflammation. The following sections cover several categories of sweeteners and their inflammatory effects.

Artificial sweeteners

Artificial, or synthetic, sweeteners are the ultimate bad guys, and for many people suffering chronic inflammation, a zero-tolerance rule is in effect here. Many artificial sweeteners, including sucralose (Splenda), are processed with solvents.

People initially saw artificial sweeteners as healthy sugar substitutes and believed these sweeteners aided in weight loss. But like alcohol, artificial sweeteners are processed through the liver — and this processing creates a level of toxicity that causes the brain to fail to recognize when the body is full. That can lead to weight gain and insulin resistance, the increasing risk for heart disease and diabetes.

When you eat something sweet, your brain gets the signal that the body is getting calories and sends a signal that the hunger is satisfied, even before the food is digested and the body knows how many calories were consumed. But when you use calorie-free artificial sweeteners, the brain can no longer use sweetness as a reliable sign of how many calories you're taking in. The brain stops sending signals of fullness, then, and you're likely to eat more.

Some of the inflammatory risks associates with some artificial sweeteners include the following:

- ✔ Heart disease
- ✔ Diabetes
- ✔ Cancer
- ✔ Increased blood pressure
- ✔ Obesity
- ✔ Neurological effects/disorders

Artificial sweeteners are used in most things listed as "diet" or "sugar free," with diet soda being a top culprit.

The best thing to do for optimum anti-inflammatory effect is to completely avoid artificial sweeteners; to satisfy a craving for something sweet, go after some fruit or a small bite of natural cocoa.

Refined sugars

Refined sugars, such as white table sugar, have been stripped down to their basic components.

The body quickly breaks refined sugar (sucrose) into the simple sugars *fructose* and *glucose*. Glucose enters the bloodstream, and cells can take in that glucose and use it for energy. Extra glucose is converted to *glycogen* and stored in the body. But when you consume too much sugar, your body has a hard time processing it all.

Because refined sugars turn to glucose quickly in your body — in other words, they're high on the *glycemic index* (see Appendix A) — they increase your risk of insulin resistance and, in turn, diabetes. Such foods create a spike in blood sugar that signals the pancreas to respond by sending out insulin in order to pull the glucose out of the blood and into the cells. The more sugary substances you eat, the harder you force your pancreas to work. You can develop diabetes as the extra sugar wears out your insulin response.

High blood sugar can also cause issues in the skin, joints, arteries, lungs, and heart. Furthermore, processing the excess sugar requires energy, and that use of energy can weaken your immune system and cause irritability and fatigue.

Table sugar isn't the only culprit. When you eat refined carbohydrates, such as white bread and white pasta, the body breaks them into sugars and processes them the same way they process table sugar.

High fructose corn syrup (HFCS) is a refined sugar that's chemically about the same thing as table sugar (sucrose) — both are about half fructose and half glucose. Some metabolic studies show that the body breaks down and uses HFCS and sucrose the same way. However, studies have also shown a link between the introduction of HFCS in the 1980s and the spike in the obesity rate in the United States. The issue may be volume — HFCS shows up everywhere.

Natural sweeteners

If you need something sweet, natural sweeteners are the best choice. A sweetener is *natural* if it comes from nature and is minimally processed or is processed without using solvents (unrefined). Natural sources tend to be easier for the body to process, lowering the risk of inflammation. They don't create a toxic reaction in the body, and most are lower on the glycemic index. You can use natural sweeteners in moderation without an appreciable risk to your health.

Here are some natural sweeteners to consider:

- ✔ **Stevia:** A product of the stevia plant, this sweetener helps treat diabetes, dermatitis, digestive problems, and hypertension. It's about 150 times sweeter than refined sugar, so you use a much smaller amount.

✔ **Honey:** Honey is rich in antioxidants and is helpful in promoting digestion, aiding with insomnia, and protecting your body against many illnesses.

✔ **Agave nectar:** Extracted from the agave plant, agave nectar is usually turned into syrup. Agave can help strengthen the immune system and fight off inflammations. Make sure you choose agave nectar that is minimally processed or raw.

✔ **Pure maple syrup:** Maple syrup helps prevent heart disease, boosts the immune system, and fights off certain cancers. You can use maple syrup as a sugar substitute in baking as well as a topping for ice cream, toast, and, of course, pancakes.

✔ **Brown rice syrup:** Brown rice syrup has a low glycemic value, which means it doesn't provide for a spike in blood sugar. It's a good source of magnesium and helps in relieving fatigue and relaxing your muscles. It's also a good source of potassium (which is good for maintaining blood pressure), iron, manganese, and B vitamins.

All the advantages of natural sweeteners don't erase the fact that you may experience some problems associated with natural sugars. Though not nearly as bad as artificial sweeteners, natural sugars still cause your blood sugar to rise. When your natural blood sugar rises too quickly or by too much, it can lead to inflammation by increasing your risk of insulin resistance and diabetes.

Low blood sugar *(hypoglycemia)* can be just as much a problem as high blood sugar *(hyperglycemia)* because too low blood sugar throws off the insulin levels, which can lead to diabetes. Therefore, the best way to consume natural sweeteners is in moderation; also choose foods on the low glycemic index and glycemic load to minimize the inflammation caused by insulin resistance and diabetes.

Balance your sweets with protein to help minimize the effect of sweet foods on your blood sugar. For example, spread some almond butter on your apple.

Eating Less Sugar

A spoonful of sugar may help the medicine go down, but most Americans don't stop at just that one spoonful. In fact, Americans on average consume 22 spoonfuls of sugar each day. Putting that number in perspective, that's about 88 grams of sugar, or the amount of sugar in four candy bars, consumed *every day.*

Nutritional guidelines for people not suffering from inflammatory diseases call for women to have no more than about 20 grams of sugar a day and for men to limit themselves to about 30 grams. People with inflammatory diseases should limit intake to natural sweeteners just once a day. If you notice a flare-up, cut out natural sweeteners completely for at least two weeks, and then bring them in again in moderation if you can't go completely without sweets.

Pinning the sugar blame on obvious culprits — candy, cookies, doughnuts, pie, soda — is easy, but sugar has a tendency to show up even where you don't suspect it. A small container of fruit-blended yogurt, for example, has about 4 spoonfuls of sugar, almost a third of the daily allowance for a woman with no dangers of inflammation.

The key to keeping sugar (and artificial sweetener) intake down is to pay attention to both nutrition labels and ingredient lists. Here are some other tips for cutting down on sugar:

- ✔ **Control portion sizes.** Sometimes a bite or two of something sweet is all you need to feel satisfied.

- ✔ **Reduce your added sugar.** Putting sugar in your coffee or tea? Gradually taper the amount you use, or try stevia in its place. When cooking, experiment with adding less sugar than the recipe calls for — you may not miss it.

- ✔ **Don't rely on food for entertainment.** When you're bored and need something to do, don't reach for the cookie jar or the candy dish. Pick up a book or call some friends or go for a walk. Celebrate achievements or special occasions with activities rather than sweets.

Giving In to Your Sweet Tooth

Sometimes you just have to say *yes* to something sweet, and that's perfectly fine as long as you do so in moderation and keep health in mind. Indulging in that little piece of dark chocolate (which is rich in antioxidants) or a small dish of fat-free yogurt topped with fresh berries feels like a better choice if you know what you're eating. In this section, we discuss both naturally sweet fruits and not-quite-so-natural baked goods.

Getting natural sugars from fruit

The best kind of sweets are the natural ones — those that look virtually the same as they did in nature. Obviously fruits top the list, and the fresher, the better. Fruit's sweetness comes from its own natural sugar, called *fructose*.

Fruit is a healthy choice, but some fruits have higher amounts of sugar than others and may still pose a risk to you when you're living with inflammation. Here are some fruits with the lowest amounts of sugar:

- Blackberries
- Cranberries
- Pears
- Raspberries
- Rhubarb

Here are some fruits with a moderate amount of sugar:

- Apples
- Cantaloupe and honeydew melons
- Grapefruit
- Papaya
- Peaches and nectarines
- Strawberries
- Watermelon

And you can find higher levels of sugar in these fruits:

- Kiwi
- Oranges
- Pineapple
- Plums

People suffering with chronic inflammation should try to limit their consumption of the following fruits, which have high levels of natural sugars:

- Bananas
- Cherries
- Dried fruit
- Grapes
- Tangerines

I'll take one of those: Finding ways to enjoy processed sweets

Ever have one of those days when a nice, gooey brownie sounds like the only thing that will make you feel better? Or when you want to skip the oatmeal and have a muffin for breakfast instead? You don't have to say *no* all the time, especially if you keep portions reasonable.

When buying sweets, try to find a bakery that uses natural or organic ingredients. If you're making the treats at home, you can use pure maple syrup or honey in place of refined white sugar — or you can experiment with adding less sugar in the first place. We discuss adjusting recipes in Chapter 16. You can also find recipes for parfaits, frozen yogurt, cookies, and even rice pudding in Chapter 15.

Part III

Enjoying Recipes for Less Inflammation and Better Health

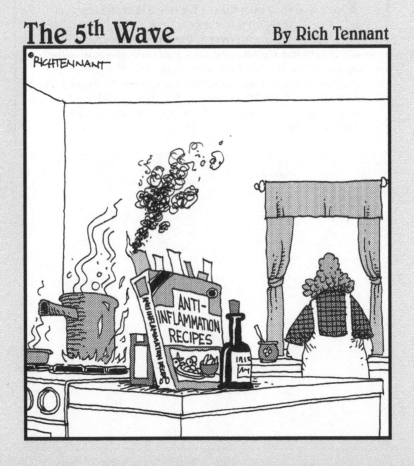

The 5th Wave By Rich Tennant

ANTI-INFLAMMATION RECIPES

In this part . . .

The best way to know for sure what you're eating is to prepare your own meals. We're excited to help you kick your cooking up a few notches (while cranking down the inflammation) with over 100 recipes in this part. We take you to the kitchen and walk you through recipes for any occasion. We help you start your day off right with unbeatable breakfasts, including smoothies. You can sample recipes for appetizers and snacks before delving into soups, salads, and entrees. We wrap up this part with tasty desserts.

Chapter 9

Starting the Day Off Right: Unbeatable Breakfasts

*Y*ou've heard it said that you never get a second chance to make a first impression. Why not use that same advice when you start each day? Getting a good start with the help of a good and good-for-you breakfast can kick-start your day with the fuel you need as well as help you fight inflammation and inflammatory conditions. Enjoying a breakfast filled with anti-inflammatory foods like nuts, berries, and flax, as well as basic fruits and vegetables, will help your body send the right signals to stop inflammation from going any farther.

The recipes in this chapter range from the simple put-it-together-and-run-out-the-door breakfasts to those that require a bit more time to complete and are suited for mornings when you have time to sit down and savor your meal.

TIP

This chapter has many recipes that call for certain kinds of fruits but also give you options to substitute fruits of your choice. When it comes to fruits and vegetables, keep in mind that organic is always best. But that rule is especially important to follow when selecting foods on the Environmental Working Group's "dirty dozen" list of produce with the highest pesticide residue: celery, peaches, strawberries, apples, domestic blueberries, nectarines, sweet bell peppers, spinach, kale, collard greens, cherries, potatoes, imported grapes, and lettuce.

Note: Many of the recipes in this chapter contain yogurt or other dairy products, which aren't great for everyone on an anti-inflammatory diet. If you have a dairy sensitivity or are lactose intolerant, good substitutes are coconut yogurt and soy yogurt.

Simple Starts: Smoothies and Yogurts

Making a smoothie in the morning is a great way to get as many vitamins, nutrients, and essentials as you can in one glass without having to make a huge meal. Smoothies aren't just good for you — they're easy. Need a quick breakfast on the go? Pour a few ingredients into a blender, blend for a few seconds, and pour. You're ready to go.

In addition to being filled with nutrients and good fats, smoothies also keep you hydrated through the morning — something you can't get with a cup of coffee. Dairy products like milk and yogurt contain a significant amount of water, so throughout the morning your body will work to pull water from those ingredients.

The live cultures in yogurt, such as acidophilus and bifidobacteria, put them in a category called *fermented foods* and help make the yogurt a dairy product that most people with lactose intolerance can tolerate. The live cultures also help keep the gastrointestinal system in top shape to fight off bacteria and pathogens, keep the immune system healthy, and keep your bowels flowing better.

A good breakfast high in nutrient-packed protein and antioxidants will balance blood sugar and protect against the inflammation that is caused by the poor regulation of blood sugar.

Making and storing flax meal

Flaxseeds are nutritionally dense and low in carbohydrates and make a great addition to many recipes, from breakfast foods to breads to soups and sauces. Flaxseeds are typically sold as whole seed, but in order to get the optimal nutritional benefit from the seeds, they should be ground into meal.

The best way to create flax meal is to simply put the seeds in a blender, food processor, or even a clean coffee grinder and process until they become a powder-like meal. They cook better and the nutritional value is strongest in this form.

In terms of storing flax meal, the oil in flax is highly unsaturated and therefore takes in oxidation quickly. That rapid oxidation can cause the meal to go rancid, rendering it useless. The best way to store flax meal is the way it's stored in nature — in the seed. When you need flax meal, grind only as much as you need and keep the rest as flaxseed. Flaxseed can be stored in a cool place for up to a year, while flax meal is good just for a few months, even if it's stored in the freezer.

Banana Coconut Milk Smoothie

Prep time: 5 min • **Cook time:** None • **Yield:** 1 serving

Ingredients	Directions
½ cup coconut milk ½ cup almond milk 1 ripe banana, peeled and sliced into ½-inch pieces 1 teaspoon cinnamon 1 tablespoon flax meal	*1* Combine the coconut milk, almond milk, banana, cinnamon, and flax meal in a blender. Blend the ingredients until smooth and pour the drink into a glass.

Per serving: Calories 463 (From Fat 297); Fat 33g (Saturated 26g); Cholesterol 0mg; Sodium 98mg; Carbohydrate 44g (Dietary Fiber 11g); Protein 6g

Tip: For more fiber and protein in your morning meal, serve this smoothie with Triple Berry Granola (see the recipe later in this chapter).

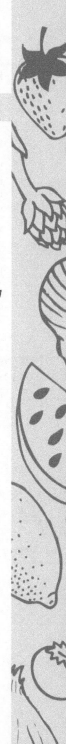

Fruit and Yogurt Parfait

Prep time: About 5 min • **Cook time:** None • **Yield:** 1 serving

Ingredients	*Directions*
1 cup plain yogurt, 0–2% fat	*1* Pour half of the yogurt into a small serving dish. Top the yogurt with half of the fruit (chopped if needed), half of the flax meal, and then half of the walnuts.
¼ cup seasonal fruit: blueberries, raspberries, bananas, strawberries, cherries, and/or peaches	
1 to 2 tablespoons flax meal	*2* Layer the remaining yogurt topped with the remaining fruit, flax meal, and walnuts.
2 tablespoons chopped walnuts	
1 to 2 tablespoons raw, unprocessed honey (optional)	*3* Drizzle with honey (if desired).

Per serving: Calories 313 (From Fat 148); Fat 17g (Saturated 4g); Cholesterol 15mg; Sodium 177mg; Carbohydrate 27g (Dietary Fiber 4g); Protein 17g

Vary It! Use your favorite flavor of nonfat Greek yogurt to give this parfait a thicker texture and richer taste.

Fruit Yogurt Drink

Prep time: 5 min • **Cook time:** None • **Yield:** 1 serving

Ingredients	Directions
1 cup plain yogurt, 0–2% fat ½ cup blueberries, fresh or frozen ¼ cup unsweetened soy-, almond, rice, oat, or hemp milk 1 tablespoon raw, unprocessed honey or ½ teaspoon stevia (optional)	*1* Combine the yogurt, blueberries, soymilk, and honey (if desired) in a blender. Blend the ingredients until smooth and pour the drink into a glass.

Per serving: Calories 215 (From Fat 47); Fat 5g (Saturated 3g); Cholesterol 15mg; Sodium 183mg; Carbohydrate 29g (Dietary Fiber 3g); Protein 15g

Vary It! Use bananas, strawberries, peaches, cherries (pits removed), or some other fruit in place of the blueberries, or combine raspberries and blackberries with the blueberries to make a mixed berry drink.

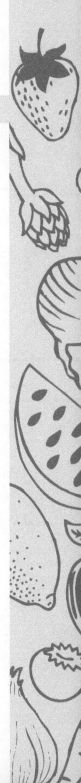

Pomegranate and Peaches with Yogurt

Prep time: 5 min • **Cook time:** None • **Yield:** 1 serving

Ingredients	*Directions*
1 cup sliced fresh peaches	**1** Arrange the peach slices in a bowl and top with the yogurt; then drizzle with the honey.
½ cup plain Greek yogurt, 0–2% fat	
1 tablespoon raw, unprocessed honey	**2** Sprinkle with the flax meal, pomegranate seeds, and almonds (if desired).
1 tablespoon flax meal	
2 tablespoons fresh pomegranate seeds	
1 teaspoon sliced almonds (optional)	

Per serving: Calories 250 (From Fat 27); Fat 3g (Saturated 0g); Cholesterol 15mg; Sodium 47mg; Carbohydrate 47g (Dietary Fiber 6g); Protein 13g

Vary It! If fresh peaches aren't in season, frozen is a good alternative for this recipe. You can also experiment with fresh or frozen organic blueberries, raspberries, cherries, or strawberries. If you use frozen fruit, just thaw it first.

Pomegranate Yogurt Cereal

Prep time: 2 min • **Cook time:** None • **Yield:** 1 serving

Ingredients	Directions
1 cup plain Greek yogurt, 0–2% fat ½ cup fresh pomegranate seeds 1 tablespoon raw, unprocessed honey 2 tablespoons whole-grain cereal, such as muesli or granola	*1* Stir together the yogurt, pomegranate seeds, and honey. Top the yogurt mixture with the whole-grain cereal.

Per serving: Calories 255 (From Fat 43); Fat 5g (Saturated 3g); Cholesterol 15mg; Sodium 92mg; Carbohydrate 36g (Dietary Fiber 1g); Protein 21g

Vary It! Replace the whole-grain cereal with homemade Triple Berry Granola (see the recipe later in this chapter).

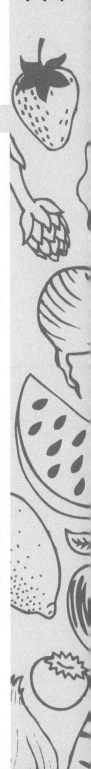

Sweetening Up Toasts, Cereals, and More

A good, healthy breakfast that is also anti-inflammatory is a great way to start your day and a perfect way to kick-start your daily fight against inflammation. Some breakfast recipes fall between the grab-n-go quick meals and the sit-down variety. They still require a bit of time in the kitchen but let you have something hearty and healthy without throwing off your morning routine.

Gluten-free breads, such as rice bread or sprouted grain bread, are packed with nutrients and higher in protein than other breads. Starting your day off with plenty of protein and whole grains keeps your blood sugar balanced, keeps your digestion running smoothly, and prevents the inflammation that is caused by blood sugar fluctuations and nutrient deficiencies.

Rice bread is typically a bit gritty, but its flavor is improved by toasting it and adding an anti-inflammatory topper, such as whole fruit spread; a spot of raw, unprocessed honey; or nut butter, such as almond butter, for an added burst of protein. (For a lunch or dinner treat, try topping it with a bit of olive oil and basil.)

When it comes to cereal, know that you have so many more options than the sugared stuff that sits on the shelves. It's true, cereal *can* be good for you. Natural grains provide antioxidants, vitamins, and nutrients your body needs.

Creating nut butters from scratch

Make nut butters to use as dips for vegetables and fruit, on toast, or in granola or yogurt. Blend 1 cup of nuts or seeds of your choice — cashews, almonds, sunflower seeds, pecans, or walnuts — or a combination of these in a blender and add a bit of olive oil as needed as it blends for the desired consistency.

When you're blending the nuts or seeds and the oil, add more olive oil to make it a bit creamier than you will actually want; nut butters must be refrigerated, which causes them to thicken a bit. If your homemade nut or seed butter starts off a bit runny, the consistency should be just about perfect once refrigerated.

You can store nut butter in the refrigerator for months. The nut butter oils will naturally separate, so stir the nut butter before using.

Pumpkin Apple Butter Toast

Prep time: 5 min • **Cook time:** 7 min • **Yield:** 1 serving

Ingredients	*Directions*
2 slices oatmeal bread	*1* Toast the oatmeal bread and spread it with the pumpkin apple butter. Sprinkle pumpkin seeds on each piece (if desired).
1 tablespoon pumpkin apple butter (see the following recipe)	
1 teaspoon pumpkin seeds, raw and unsalted (optional)	

Per serving: Calories 150 (From Fat 22); Fat 2g (Saturated 0g); Cholesterol 0mg; Sodium 326mg; Carbohydrate 27g (Dietary Fiber 2g); Protein 5g

Pumpkin Apple Butter

1 cup cooked pumpkin or an 8-ounce can of organic pumpkin	*1* Combine the pumpkin, apple juice, ginger, and cinnamon in a small saucepan. Cook the mixture over medium heat, whisking constantly, about 5 minutes or until it reaches a good spreading consistency.
2 tablespoons apple juice	
1 teaspoon ground ginger	
1 teaspoon cinnamon	

Per serving: Calories 5 (From Fat 0); Fat 0g (Saturated 0g); Cholesterol 0mg; Sodium 0mg; Carbohydrate 1g (Dietary Fiber 0g); Protein 0g per tbsp

Tip: If you use fresh cooked pumpkin, it may need more cooking time to achieve the desired spreadable consistency.

Note: You may keep Pumpkin Apple Butter in the refrigerator for up to one week.

Cashew Butter and Banana Toast

Prep time: 5 min • **Cook time:** 2 min • **Yield:** 2 servings

Ingredients	*Directions*
½ cup unsalted roasted cashews	*1* Combine the cashews and the salt in a small food processor; puree until smooth.
Dash salt	
2 slices oat or rice bread	*2* Toast the two pieces of bread and spread them with the cashew mixture.
1 ripe banana, peeled and sliced	
Pinch of cinnamon	*3* Add sliced banana to the toast and sprinkle it with the cinnamon and flax meal. Drizzle the toast with honey.
1 teaspoon flax meal	
1 teaspoon raw, unprocessed honey	

Per serving: *Calories 334 (From Fat 157); Fat 18g (Saturated 3g); Cholesterol 0mg; Sodium 1,331mg; Carbohydrate 40g (Dietary Fiber 4g); Protein 9g*

Rice Bread with Apricot Yogurt

Prep time: 5 min • **Cook time:** None • **Yield:** 1 serving

Ingredients	Directions
¼ cup plain Greek yogurt, 0–2% fat	**1** Stir together the yogurt, apricots, honey, and cinnamon.
1 fresh or 2 dried apricots, cut into pieces	**2** Toast the bread and spread the yogurt mixture on each slice.
2 tablespoons raw, unprocessed honey (optional)	
1 teaspoon cinnamon	
2 slices rice bread	

Per serving: Calories 182 (From Fat 33); Fat 4g (Saturated 1g); Cholesterol 4mg; Sodium 237mg; Carbohydrate 30g (Dietary Fiber 5g); Protein 10g

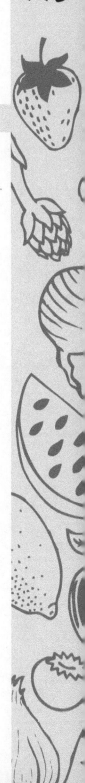

Nutty Steel-Cut Oats

Prep time: 5 min • **Cook time:** 10–30 min • **Yield:** 1 serving

Ingredients	*Directions*
4 cups water	*1* In a medium saucepan, boil the water. Add the oats, reduce the heat to low, and simmer for 10 to 30 minutes until they reach the desired doneness.
1 cup steel-cut oats	
1 to 2 tablespoons flax meal	
¼ cup mixed raw nuts, such as cashews and almonds	*2* Stir the flax meal, nuts, milk, and berries into the oats. Drizzle honey across the top if desired. Serve hot.
2 tablespoons unsweetened almond, rice, or hemp milk	
2 tablespoons thawed frozen or fresh blueberries	
1 to 2 tablespoons raw, unprocessed honey or agave nectar, or ½ teaspoon stevia (optional)	

Per serving: Calories 927 (From Fat 293); Fat 33g (Saturated 3g); Cholesterol 0mg; Sodium 39mg; Carbohydrate 140g (Dietary Fiber 22g); Protein 32g

Tip: In order to get the health benefits of oatmeal for breakfast, it's important not to overcook the oats. The longer they cook, the more their starches break down.

Hot Brown Rice Cereal

Prep time: 5 min • **Cook time:** 10 min • **Yield:** 1 serving

Ingredients	*Directions*
½ cup uncooked brown rice 1 cup water ¼ cup chopped walnuts 2 tablespoons flax meal Seasonal fruit, such as blueberries, cherries, raspberries, or apples, chopped as needed	*1* In a medium skillet over medium heat, toast the brown rice, stirring constantly, until the rice is slightly brown, about 5 to 7 minutes. Remove from the heat and let the rice cool. *2* Grind the rice in a food processor until it becomes powdered. *3* Boil the water in a medium saucepan and add the powdered rice. Reduce the heat to a simmer. Continue stirring the rice mixture until it's thick, about 7 minutes. *4* Stir in the walnuts, flax meal, and fruit. Serve hot.

Per serving: Calories 642 (From Fat 253); Fat 28g (Saturated 3g); Cholesterol 0mg; Sodium 22mg; Carbohydrate 86g (Dietary Fiber 14g); Protein 16g

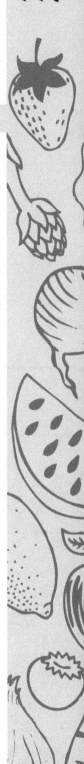

Triple Berry Granola

Prep time: 10 min • **Cook time:** About 1 hr • **Yield:** 6 cups

Ingredients	Directions
5 cups rolled oats	*1* Preheat the oven to 250 degrees.
1 cup raw almonds	
3 tablespoons flax meal	*2* In a large bowl, combine the oats, almonds, flax meal, and sea salt; set the mixture aside.
½ teaspoon sea salt	
1 cup agave nectar	*3* Combine the agave nectar, vanilla extract, cinnamon, and sesame oil in a small bowl. Stir this mixture into the dry ingredients and mix well.
2 tablespoons real vanilla extract	
2 tablespoons cinnamon	*4* Smooth the granola mixture onto a baking sheet and bake for about an hour, stirring often to cook evenly and prevent the granola from burning. While the granola bakes, thaw, rinse, and strain the mixed berries.
½ cup cold-pressed sesame oil	
1½ cups frozen mixed berries (strawberries, blueberries, and raspberries)	*5* Remove the granola from the pan and place it in a large bowl. Stir the berries into the granola and enjoy 1 cup servings.

Per serving: Calories 771 (From Fat 330); Fat 37g (Saturated 5g); Cholesterol 0mg; Sodium 204mg; Carbohydrate 99g (Dietary Fiber 16g); Protein 17g

Tip: Serve the granola with almond milk for a granola breakfast cereal, or use the granola as a topping for plain yogurt.

Note: The granola can be stored in the refrigerator for up to one week with fresh fruit added or in the pantry for up to one month if you omit the fruit.

Gluten-free Banana Breakfast Bars

Prep time: 10 min • **Cook time:** 25 min • **Yield:** 12 bars

Ingredients	Directions
½ cup coconut oil, room temperature, divided	**1** Preheat the oven to 425 degrees. Grease a 9-x13-inch baking pan with 1 teaspoon of the coconut oil.
1¼ cups brown rice flour	
¼ cup arrowroot flour	**2** In a small bowl, sift together the flours, flax meal, baking soda, salt, cardamom, and cinnamon. Set these dry ingredients aside.
1 tablespoon flax meal	
½ teaspoon baking soda	
1 teaspoon sea salt	**3** In a large bowl, beat together the remaining coconut oil, the wheat germ oil, the stevia, and the egg. Add the bananas and vanilla, and keep beating the mixture until it's smooth.
½ teaspoon ground cardamom	
1 teaspoon cinnamon	
1 tablespoon wheat germ oil	
1 cup stevia	**4** Add the flour mixture as well as the oats and nuts (if desired) to the wet ingredients, and stir until the batter is evenly mixed. Pour the batter into the greased baking pan.
1 egg	
3 medium ripe bananas, mashed	
1 teaspoon vanilla	**5** Bake the bars until golden, approximately 25 minutes. Cut into 12 squares.
1½ cups raw, quick-cooking oats	
¾ cup sliced almonds (optional)	

Per serving: Calories 185 (From Fat 105); Fat 12g (Saturated 8g); Cholesterol 18mg; Sodium 250mg; Carbohydrate 19g (Dietary Fiber 3g); Protein 3g

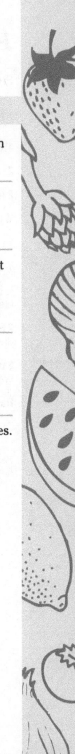

Pumpkin Apple Butter Pancakes

Prep time: 15 min • **Cook time:** 20 min • **Yield:** 3–4 servings

Ingredients	*Directions*
1¼ cups buckwheat flour 2 tablespoons tapioca flour 2 teaspoons baking powder ½ teaspoon sea salt 1 egg, beaten ½ cup plain yogurt, 0–2% fat ½ cup pumpkin apple butter (see the following recipe) 2 tablespoons coconut oil, divided 2 tablespoons chopped walnuts (optional) Dark maple syrup (optional)	**1** Combine the flours, baking powder, and salt in a medium bowl. **2** Add the yogurt and pumpkin apple butter to the beaten egg, and then add these wet ingredients to the dry mixture. **3** Warm a large skillet over low to medium heat, and then add about 2 teaspoons of coconut oil. Drop 2 tablespoons of pancake batter in the oil and cook on both sides until golden brown. Flip the pancakes when you see bubbles rising to the surface. **4** Repeat Step 3 with the remaining coconut oil and pancake batter. **5** Top with walnuts and maple syrup (if desired).

Per serving: Calories 324 (From Fat 123); Fat 14g (Saturated 10g); Cholesterol 76mg; Sodium 683mg; Carbohydrate 45g (Dietary Fiber 6g); Protein 10g

Pumpkin Apple Butter

1 cup cooked pumpkin or an 8-ounce can of organic pumpkin

2 tablespoons apple juice

1 teaspoon ground ginger

1 teaspoon cinnamon

1 Combine the pumpkin, apple juice, ginger, and cinnamon in a small saucepan. Cook the mixture over medium heat, whisking constantly, about 5 minutes or until it reaches a good spreading consistency.

Per serving: Calories 5 (From Fat 0); Fat 0g (Saturated 0g); Cholesterol 0mg; Sodium 0mg; Carbohydrate 1g (Dietary Fiber 0g); Protein 0g per tbsp

Tip: If you use fresh cooked pumpkin, it may need more cooking time to achieve the desired spreadable consistency.

Note: You may keep Pumpkin Apple Butter in the refrigerator for up to one week.

Tip: For a dairy-free option, substitute ½ cup coconut milk for the yogurt.

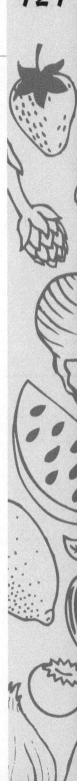

Enjoying Savory Egg Breakfasts

Sometimes breakfast should be savored. Eggs are a great way to start off the day with a protein- and nutrient-dense super food. A hearty breakfast that includes eggs can keep you fuller longer and eliminate the need for a lot of snacking through the day. An added benefit is that, for most people, eggs are anti-inflammatory. In fact, people who eat a steady breakfast of eggs, fresh fruit, and a cup of coffee can reduce their inflammation markers by up to 20 percent.

We recommend you eat up to four omega-3-enriched eggs per week, and be sure to use the whole egg. Don't skimp on the yolk, because that is where a lot of the anti-inflammatory benefit is found in the form of vitamin D and choline, a fat that helps support brain health and decreases C-reactive protein (CRP).

Any food can trigger a food sensitivity if you eat too much of it, so don't exceed the four eggs per week recommendation.

Choose organic, free-range, or pastured eggs. Eggs from chickens that have been feeding on grass, called pastured eggs or free-range, have a higher omega-3 content because of what the animals eat. If you're feeling ambitious, you can "grow" your own eggs by keeping your own chickens on your property. Contact your local cooperative extension office for more details or regulations on this practice, and check out *Raising Chickens For Dummies* by Kimberly Willis and Rob Ludlow (Wiley).

Poached Eggs with Spinach and Swiss Chard

Prep time: 5 min • **Cook time:** 5 min • **Yield:** 2 servings

Ingredients	Directions
2 eggs	*1* Bring 2 cups of water to near boiling in a shallow pan. Crack one egg into a small bowl, lower the bowl almost to the water, and pour the egg into the water. Repeat with the other egg.
2 slices oat or rice bread	
½ teaspoon extra-virgin olive oil	
10 fresh baby spinach leaves	*2* Use a teaspoon to nudge the egg whites closer to the yolk, helping to keep the egg whites together. Then let the eggs poach untouched for about 3 to 4 minutes. Lift the eggs out of the water gently, one at a time, with a slotted spoon, and place them on a plate.
10 Swiss chard leaves	
2 tablespoons chopped fresh parsley	
Sea salt to taste	*3* Toast the bread while you lightly sauté the spinach and Swiss chard in olive oil in a small sauté pan for 5 to 7 minutes.
Freshly ground pepper to taste	
Dried mint to taste	
	4 Use the sautéed greens and parsley to make a bed of greens on the toasted bread.
	5 Add the poached eggs to the bed of greens. Sprinkle the eggs with sea salt, ground pepper, and dried mint to taste.

Per serving: Calories 164 (From Fat 67); Fat 7g (Saturated 2g); Cholesterol 213mg; Sodium 558mg; Carbohydrate 15g (Dietary Fiber 2g); Protein 9g

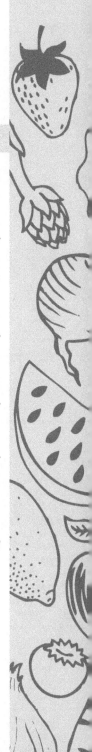

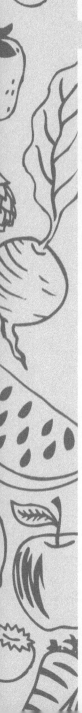

Fresh Vegetable Frittata

Prep time: 5 min • **Cook time:** 15 min • **Yield:** 1–2 servings

Ingredients	*Directions*
4 teaspoons extra-virgin olive oil **2 tablespoons chopped onions** **½ cup chopped seasonal fresh vegetables, such as zucchini, asparagus, spinach, broccoli, and kale, chopped** **3 eggs, beaten well with a splash of water** **1 tablespoon goat cheese (optional)**	*1* Heat the olive oil in a medium nonstick skillet over medium heat. Sauté the onions in the olive oil until they're slightly translucent, about 5 minutes. Add the remaining vegetables and sauté for a few minutes until slightly softened. *2* Pour the beaten eggs into the vegetable mixture and cook 5 to 7 minutes until the egg is set. Push the cooked egg into the center of the pan, letting the raw egg move to the edges of the pan. *3* Slide the frittata onto a plate and top with goat cheese (if desired).

Per serving: Calories 399 (From Fat 298); Fat 33g (Saturated 7g); Cholesterol 638mg; Sodium 192mg; Carbohydrate 5g (Dietary Fiber 1g); Protein 20g

Tip: Pair this frittata with oat or rice toast for a full two servings.

Mushroom Omelet with Dill

Prep time: 5 min • **Cook time:** 15 min • **Yield:** 1 serving

Ingredients	*Directions*
4 teaspoons extra-virgin olive oil	*1* Heat the olive oil in a medium nonstick skillet over medium heat. Sauté the onions and garlic until they're translucent, about 5 minutes. Add the mushrooms and continue to sauté until the mushrooms are soft, about 10 minutes. Set the mushroom mixture aside in a separate bowl.
2 tablespoons chopped sweet onion	
1 clove garlic, chopped	
1 cup sliced mushrooms	
2 eggs, beaten well with a splash of water	*2* Add a splash of olive oil to the skillet you used to sauté the mushrooms, and add the egg. Push the cooked egg into the center of the pan, letting the raw egg move to the edges of the pan. After about 5 minutes, spoon the mushroom mixture onto one side of the omelet.
2 tablespoons unprocessed cheddar, Swiss, or soy cheese, or hard goat cheese (optional)	
3 tablespoons chopped fresh dill	*3* Sprinkle the omelet with the cheese (if desired) and dill. Fold the plain egg over the side with the mushrooms and continue to cook for about 3 to 5 minutes, to firm up the inside of the omelet. Slide the omelet onto a plate and serve.

Per serving: *Calories 339 (From Fat 255); Fat 28g (Saturated 6g); Cholesterol 425mg; Sodium 132mg; Carbohydrate 7g (Dietary Fiber 1g); Protein 15g*

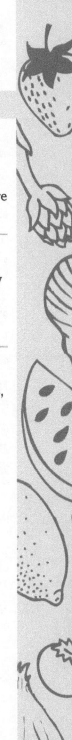

Broccoli and Red Pepper Quiche

Prep time: 20 min • **Cook time:** 1 hr, 10 min • **Yield:** 6 servings

Ingredients	Directions
8- or 9-inch frozen whole-wheat pie crust	**1** Preheat the oven to 400 degrees. Thaw the frozen pie shell for 10 minutes at room temperature, and then prick the bottom with a fork.
Olive oil cooking spray	
2 tablespoons extra-virgin olive oil	**2** Spray a piece of aluminum foil with olive oil cooking spray and lay it in the bottom of the shell; weigh down the foil with rice or dried beans. Bake the pie shell for 10 minutes or until it's golden. Remove the pie shell from the oven and reduce the oven temperature to 350 degrees.
½ small onion, diced	
2 tablespoons chopped broccoli	
½ red bell pepper, seeded and chopped	**3** Heat the olive oil in a medium skillet over medium heat. Sauté the onions in the olive oil until they're translucent, about 5 minutes. Add the broccoli and red bell pepper. Sauté until they're soft, about 10 to 12 minutes.
1 cup coconut milk	
4 eggs	
1 tablespoon dried oregano	**4** In a medium bowl, combine the coconut milk, eggs, oregano, nutmeg, ground pepper, and salt. Whisk in the vegetable mixture, and pour into the pie shell.
⅛ teaspoon nutmeg	
¼ teaspoon freshly ground pepper	
⅛ teaspoon sea salt	**5** Bake the quiche in the center of the oven for approximately 45 minutes or until the center is set and is firm when you jiggle the pan.

Per serving: Calories 357 (From Fat 281); Fat 31g (Saturated 15g); Cholesterol 142mg; Sodium 256mg; Carbohydrate 15g (Dietary Fiber 4g); Protein 8g

Note: You can store this quiche in the refrigerator for up to three days.

Tip: If you have gluten sensitivities, replace the pie crust with a mixture of ½ cup cooked quinoa and 1 teaspoon olive oil, pressed into a pie plate.

Chapter 10

Something on the Side: Appetizers and Snacks

In This Chapter

▶ Making healthy dips and cheesy snacks

▶ Getting your omega-3s with seafood appetizers

▶ Fixing appetizers with good fillings

▶ Finding easy ways to snack

*J*ust because you're on an anti-inflammatory diet doesn't mean your menu has to be bland and boring. What if you could include smoked salmon, spicy ground turkey, and baked Brie cheese to your list of options? In this chapter, we introduce quick and easy snacks and appetizers as well as those you'd be proud to break out when entertaining at home. Not only do these recipes feature beans and nuts, vegetables and fruits, and seafood and soft cheeses, but they also contain some anti-inflammatory powerhouses in the form of fresh herbs and spices. You can satisfy your taste buds and fight inflammation with the garlic, turmeric, cayenne, basil, cilantro, parsley, black pepper, and more you see here.

Making Dips Everyone Enjoys

Ask anyone, and they'll likely tell you the same thing: The center of attention at the food table for any gathering is a good bowl of dip. That bowl of creamy goodness may seem like a good idea, but it's what's lurking under the surface that can really get you down.

Many creamy dips are made with mayonnaise and high-fat cheese — two things you'll want to stay away from with an anti-inflammatory diet. However, most of those dips can be made using healthy alternatives that keep them good tasting but also good for you.

Swap plain lowfat yogurt or lowfat or no-fat cream cheese — or better yet, nondairy or soy cheese — for mayonnaise. Toss a mashed avocado into the mix to pack your dip with good fats and help to decrease bad cholesterol and increase good cholesterol. (Figure 10-1 shows you how to pit an avocado.) Or create a creamy bean dip by putting cooked beans through your blender or food processor before adding a bit of flavor and flair with fresh herbs, such as dill, thyme, or basil.

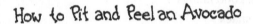

How to Pit and Peel an Avocado

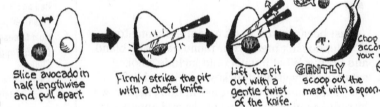

Figure 10-1:
Pitting an avocado.

Slice avocado in half lengthwise and pull apart.

Firmly strike the pit with a chef's knife.

Lift the pit out with a gentle twist of the knife.

GENTLY scoop out the meat with a spoon.

Chop or slice according to your recipe.

Healthy alternatives to corn chips with any dip or salsa include celery stalks, whole-grain chips, or crackers or organic flatbreads.

Avocado and Black Bean Dip

Prep time: 15 min • **Cook time:** None • **Yield:** 6 servings

Ingredients	*Directions*
15-ounces canned black beans, rinsed	*1* Combine the black beans, tomatoes, scallions, lemon juice, and cilantro. Add the avocado and mix well. Add black pepper, sea salt, and cayenne pepper to taste.
½ cup chopped tomatoes	
1 small scallion, chopped	
2 tablespoons fresh lemon juice	*2* Serve the dip with corn chips or whole-grain chips.
2 tablespoons chopped fresh cilantro	
1 avocado, peeled, pitted, and chopped	
Freshly ground black pepper to taste	
Sea salt to taste	
½ teaspoon cayenne pepper, or to taste	
Corn chips or whole-grain chips for serving	

Per serving: Calories 92 (From Fat 42); Fat 5g (Saturated 1g); Cholesterol 0mg; Sodium 183mg; Carbohydrate 10g (Dietary Fiber 5g); Protein 4g

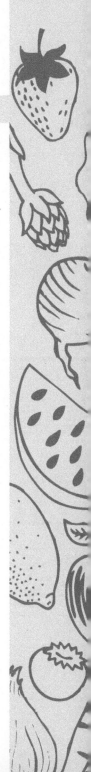

Avocado and Chickpea Guacamole

Prep time: 15 min • **Cook time:** None • **Yield:** 4 servings

Ingredients	*Directions*
2 ripe avocados	*1* Peel, pit, and mash the avocados with the back of a fork or a potato masher in a medium bowl.
¼ cup chickpeas	
1 small onion	*2* Pulse the chickpeas in a food processor until they reach the desired consistency, and then add to the avocados.
1 small serrano chile, or to taste	
2 tablespoons chopped fresh cilantro	*3* Finely chop the onion and serrano chile. Add the onions, serrano chile, cilantro, and parsley to the avocado and chickpea mixture. Mix in the lemon juice and sea salt.
1 tablespoon chopped fresh parsley	
Juice of 1 lemon	
Sea salt to taste	*4* Serve with celery sticks or rice crackers.
Celery sticks or rice crackers for serving	

Per serving: Calories 148 (From Fat 113); Fat 13g (Saturated 3g); Cholesterol 0mg; Sodium 145mg; Carbohydrate 10g (Dietary Fiber 8g); Protein 3g

Artichoke Dip

Prep time: 10 min • **Cook time:** 3–5 min • **Yield:** 4 servings

Ingredients	*Directions*
¼ cup grated mozzarella cheese or dairy-free cheese (optional)	*1* Adjust the oven rack so the food will be about four inches from the upper heating element. Turn on the broiler.
½ teaspoon chopped garlic	
2 cups marinated artichokes, chopped	*2* Combine the cheese (if desired) and garlic in a medium bowl.
2 tablespoons reserved artichoke marinade	*3* Add the artichokes and 2 tablespoons artichoke marinade, and mix well.
2 tablespoons chopped parsley	
Rice crackers or pita bread for serving	*4* Spoon the mixture into an oven-safe glass or ceramic pie plate. Broil uncovered for 3 to 5 minutes or until the artichokes are soft.
	5 Top with chopped parsley, and serve with rice crackers or pita bread.

Per serving: Calories 65 (From Fat 16); Fat 2g (Saturated 1g); Cholesterol 6mg; Sodium 295mg; Carbohydrate 9g (Dietary Fiber 0g); Protein 4g

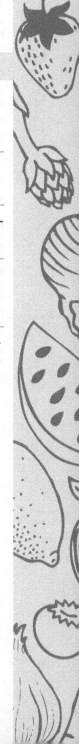

White Bean Dip

Prep time: 15 min • **Cook time:** None • **Yield:** 6 servings

Ingredients	*Directions*
8 ounces canned white beans (cannellini beans)	*1* Combine the white beans, garlic, olive oil, lemon juice, and sage in a food processor. Pulse the mixture until it's blended. Season with salt and black pepper to taste. Mix well.
2 cloves garlic	
5 tablespoons extra-virgin olive oil	
Juice of 1 lemon	*2* Serve with rice crackers or whole-grain pita bread.
1 teaspoon dried sage	
Sea salt to taste	
Freshly ground black pepper to taste	
Rice crackers or pita bread for serving	

Per serving: Calories 133 (From Fat 103); Fat 11g (Saturated 2g); Cholesterol 0mg; Sodium 175mg; Carbohydrate 6g (Dietary Fiber 2g); Protein 2g

Nutty Hummus Dip

Prep time: 10 min • **Cook time:** None • **Yield:** 8 servings

Ingredients	*Directions*
2 cups cooked chickpeas	**1** Combine the chickpeas, walnuts, garlic, lemon juice, olive oil, and parsley in a food processor and pulse until smooth. Season the dip with salt and pepper to taste. Mix well.
2 tablespoons walnut pieces	
4 cloves garlic	
Juice of 2 lemons	
2 tablespoons extra-virgin olive oil	**2** Serve with organic baby carrots, celery sticks, or whole-grain pita strips for dipping.
1 tablespoon dried parsley	
Sea salt to taste	
Freshly ground pepper to taste	
Organic baby carrots, celery sticks, or whole-grain pita strips for serving	

Per serving: Calories 115 (From Fat 51); Fat 6g (Saturated 1g); Cholesterol 0mg; Sodium 76mg; Carbohydrate 13g (Dietary Fiber 3g); Protein 4g

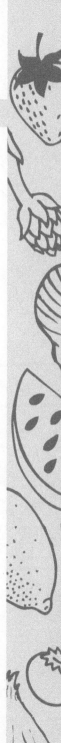

Red and Green Salsa

Prep time: 10 min • **Cook time:** None • **Yield:** 6 servings

Ingredients	*Directions*
2 large tomatoes, chopped	*1* Combine the chopped tomatoes, onion, avocado, serrano chile, cilantro, and parsley in a medium bowl.
¼ cup chopped red onion	
1 large avocado, peeled, pitted, and chopped	*2* Squeeze the lime juice into the mixture and sprinkle with sea salt to taste. Gently mix.
1 small serrano chile, or to taste, finely chopped	
2 tablespoons chopped fresh cilantro	*3* Serve with rice crackers.
1 tablespoon chopped parsley	
Splash of fresh lime juice	
Sea salt to taste	
Rice crackers for serving	

Per serving: Calories 67 (From Fat 47); Fat 5g (Saturated 1g); Cholesterol 0mg; Sodium 106mg; Carbohydrate 6g (Dietary Fiber 2g); Protein 1g

Note: This recipe contains members of the nightshade family — green peppers and tomatoes — which may cause inflammation for some people.

Choosing Soft Cheeses for Cheesy Appetizers

Cheese is a dairy product that can contain a considerable amount of fat, calories, and carbohydrates per serving; however, when you choose the right types of cheeses and eat them in moderation, cheese is a delicious source of calcium and nutrients.

Different types of cheeses are tolerated differently by different people. For example, some people can tolerate sheep's milk or goat's milk cheeses, such as feta cheese or Gouda made with goat's milk. Other people suffer no inflammation or ill effects from cow's milk cheeses, such as mozzarella and cheddar. Food sensitivity and constitution are factors in determining which types of cheeses are okay for you.

Choose the lower-fat version so that the fat content doesn't contribute to weight gain, and also choose unprocessed cheese. Processed cheeses are inflammatory because they can contain additives, preservatives, and chemicals that act as food toxins or create inflammation in the body.

Signs of cheese and dairy products causing inflammation include runny nose, sinus congestion, fatigue, bloating, and gas. If dairy products are a problem for you, substitute traditional cheeses with soy- or rice-based "cheeses" that you can find at your health food store.

Feta Cheese Plate

Prep time: 5 min • **Cook time:** None • **Yield:** 4 servings

Ingredients	*Directions*
4–6 ounces feta cheese in bite-sized pieces **1 tablespoon extra-virgin olive oil** **1 teaspoon crushed fresh mint leaves**	*1* Drizzle the feta cheese with olive oil, and then sprinkle it with crushed mint leaves. Serve the feta with small forks or toothpicks.

Per serving: Calories 105 (From Fat 85); Fat 9g (Saturated 5g); Cholesterol 25mg; Sodium 317mg; Carbohydrate 1g (Dietary Fiber 0g); Protein 4g

Goat Cheese Bruschetta

Prep time: 10 min • **Cook time:** 2 to 5 min • **Yield:** 6 servings

Ingredients	*Directions*
Fresh whole-grain French bread, sliced into twelve 1-inch slices	*1* Preheat the oven to 400 degrees.
1 large tomato, finely diced	*2* Combine the goat cheese and the tomato in a small bowl.
½ cup goat cheese	
6 teaspoons Parmesan cheese	*3* Top each slice of bread with at least 1 tablespoon of the tomato mixture. Sprinkle each slice with a teaspoon of Parmesan cheese.
3 tablespoons fresh basil leaves	
	4 Bake the slices for 2 to 5 minutes or until they're slightly golden. Top each slice with a basil leaf and serve.

Per serving: Calories 142 (From Fat 52); Fat 6g (Saturated 3g); Cholesterol 10mg; Sodium 254mg; Carbohydrate 16g (Dietary Fiber 2g); Protein 8g

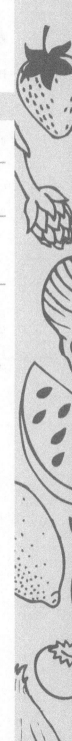

Ginger-Topped Goat Cheese

Prep time: 5 min • **Cook time:** 10 min • **Yield:** 6 servings

Ingredients	*Directions*
8-ounce goat cheese log	**1** Preheat the oven to 350 degrees.
3 tablespoons ginger syrup	
¼ cup pecans	**2** Place the goat cheese log in a small, ovenproof baking dish. Coat the top of the cheese with ginger syrup and arrange the pecans on top of the syrup.
Rice crackers for serving	
	3 Bake the goat cheese until it's soft and the pecans are lightly toasted, approximately 10 minutes. Serve with crackers.

Per serving: Calories 157 (From Fat 101); Fat 11g (Saturated 6g); Cholesterol 17mg; Sodium 145mg; Carbohydrate 8g (Dietary Fiber 1g); Protein 7g

Tip: Head to Chapter 15 for the ginger syrup recipe. (For thicker ginger syrup, add 1 package powdered pectin to the syrup while cooking according to the recipe in Chapter 15.)

Whipping Up Seafood Starters

Nutrition experts and dietitians may disagree on a variety of things, but one thing they agree on is that seafood should be a regular part of your weekly menu.

Deep-sea fish contain a high amount of omega-3 fatty acids — the essential fats that your body isn't capable of making on its own. Those omega-3 fatty acids are a mighty bunch, effective in fighting cancer, heart disease, and arthritis.

The recipe for Baked Crab Rangoon uses wonton wrappers to contain the filling. Figure 10-2 shows you how to wrap your apps.

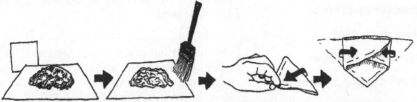

Figure 10-2:
Folding
wontons.

PLACE 1 HEAPING
TEASPOON OF FILLING
IN THE CENTER OF
THE WRAPPER.

BRUSH THE EDGES OF THE
WRAPPER WITH THE BEA-
TEN EGG.

FOLD THE WRAPPER IN
HALF TO FORM A TRIANGLE.
PINCH EDGES TO SEAL.

PULL 2 OPPOSITE
CORNERS TOGETHER.
MOISTEN ONE CORNER
WITH EGG. OVERLAP
WITH OTHER CORNER
PRESS TO SEAL.

FOLDING WONTONS

Vietnamese Spring Rolls

Prep time: 20 min • **Cook time:** None • **Yield:** 6 servings

Ingredients	*Directions*
½ **cup diced cooked chicken breast, salmon, or firm tofu**	*1* Mix the meat or tofu and cucumber in a medium bowl. Add the rice wine vinegar, lime juice, agave nectar, and sea salt. Mix until combined.
½ **cup finely sliced cucumber**	
1 tablespoon rice wine vinegar	*2* Dip one rice paper wrapper in warm water and lay flat on a clean, dry surface. Place a few leaves of spinach in the center of the wrapper, and then add a dollop of the meat or tofu mixture, a few slices of avocado, and three cilantro leaves.
2 teaspoons fresh lime juice	
1 teaspoon agave nectar	
½ **teaspoon sea salt**	
12 rice paper wrappers	*3* Fold the bottom of the rice paper over the mixture, then fold in the sides, and roll tightly. Place the roll on a plate and repeat with the remaining rice papers and filling. Serve with dipping sauce.
½ **cup baby spinach leaves**	
1 avocado, peeled, pitted, and finely sliced	
36 leaves fresh cilantro	
Dipping sauce (see the following recipe)	

Dipping sauce

5 tablespoons wheat-free tamari sauce	*1* Mix the tamari sauce, lime juice, rice wine vinegar, chili paste, and cilantro in a small bowl. Dip the shrimp rolls or drizzle the sauce over them with a small spoon.
1 teaspoon fresh lime juice	
2 teaspoons rice wine vinegar	
1 teaspoon chili paste	
1 teaspoon chopped fresh cilantro	

Per serving: Calories 121 (From Fat 44); Fat 5g (Saturated 1g); Cholesterol 10mg; Sodium 1,011mg; Carbohydrate 12g (Dietary Fiber 3g); Protein 8g

Spicy Oysters on the Shell

Prep time: 8 min • **Cook time:** None • **Yield:** 6 servings

Ingredients	*Directions*
4 ounces tomato juice	*1* Mix the tomato juice, horseradish, juice of one lemon, and crushed red pepper in a small bowl.
1 teaspoon horseradish	
2 lemons	
1 teaspoon crushed red pepper	*2* Drizzle the tomato mixture over the oysters. Serve with the other lemon cut into lemon wedges.
10 ounces raw oysters, well-cleaned and cut on the half shell	

Per serving: Calories 42 (From Fat 12); Fat 1g (Saturated 0g); Cholesterol 25mg; Sodium 170mg; Carbohydrate 4g (Dietary Fiber 0g); Protein 4g

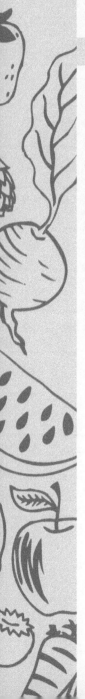

Skewered Shrimp with Lemon and Garlic

Prep time: 15 min • **Cook time:** None • **Yield:** 6 servings

Ingredients	*Directions*
3 tablespoons minced garlic	*1* Combine the garlic, olive oil, lemon juice, parsley, salt, black pepper, and shrimp in a medium bowl. Toss together.
2 tablespoons extra-virgin olive oil	
¼ cup fresh lemon juice	
¼ cup minced fresh parsley	*2* Serve the shrimp on skewers, sprinkled with the crumbled feta cheese (if desired) and with pita chips on the side.
½ teaspoon sea salt	
½ teaspoon freshly ground black pepper	
1¼ pounds cooked shrimp, shelled and deveined	
¼ cup crumbled feta cheese (optional)	
Pita chips for serving	

Per serving: Calories 144 (From Fat 50); Fat 6g (Saturated 1g); Cholesterol 184mg; Sodium 406mg; Carbohydrate 3g (Dietary Fiber 0g); Protein 20g

Baked Crab Rangoon

Prep time: 15 min • **Cook time:** 20 min • **Yield:** 12 servings

Ingredients	Directions
8 ounces fat-free cream cheese or soy cheese spread	**1** Preheat the oven to 350 degrees. Combine the cream cheese or soy cheese, crab meat, scallions, Worcestershire sauce, soy sauce, and garlic in a bowl. Mix well and season with black pepper to taste.
8 ounces fresh or canned crab meat, drained and flaked	
2 scallions, finely chopped	**2** Lay a wonton wrapper on a flat surface and wet the edges with a little water. Add 1 teaspoon of crab filling to the middle of the wrapper; fold over the edges of the wrapper to make a triangle shape. Wet the edges and press them together to seal.
½ teaspoon Worcestershire sauce	
½ teaspoon soy sauce	
1 large clove garlic, finely chopped	**3** Keep the crab rangoon covered with a damp paper towel to keep them from drying out while you repeat Step 2 with the rest of the wrappers and filling.
12 wonton wrappers	
Freshly ground black pepper to taste	**4** Arrange the crab rangoon on a medium-sized baking sheet brushed with sesame oil. Brush the surface of the crab rangoon with sesame oil.
Sesame oil	
Sweet and sour sauce (optional)	**5** Bake the crab rangoon for 10 minutes and then flip them over. Bake for another 10 minutes or until they're slightly golden brown.
	6 Serve the crab rangoon hot with sweet and sour sauce (if desired).

Per serving: Calories 114 (From Fat 84); Fat 9g (Saturated 4g); Cholesterol 32mg; Sodium 224mg; Carbohydrate 6g (Dietary Fiber 0g); Protein 5g

Smoked Salmon Bites

Prep time: 10 min • **Cook time:** None • **Yield:** 6 servings

Ingredients	Directions
4 ounces spreadable goat cheese or soy cheese spread	**1** Combine the cheese, dill, and smoked salmon in a food processor. Puree until smooth.
2 tablespoons chopped fresh dill	
8 ounces North Atlantic smoked salmon	**2** Add black pepper to taste and mix well. Serve with savory rice crackers.
Fresh ground black pepper to taste	
Rice crackers for serving	

Per serving: Calories 95 (From Fat 51); Fat 6g (Saturated 3g); Cholesterol 17mg; Sodium 826mg; Carbohydrate 0g (Dietary Fiber 0g); Protein 10g

Smoked Salmon and Asparagus Rolls

Prep time: 10 min • **Cook time:** 2–5 min • **Yield:** 6 servings

Ingredients	Directions
8 ounces North Atlantic smoked salmon	**1** Lightly steam the asparagus spears in a covered saucepan with water for 2 to 5 minutes. Let the asparagus cool.
12 asparagus spears	
Juice of 1 lemon	**2** Wrap a piece of smoked salmon around each asparagus spear. Sprinkle the spears with lemon juice, chopped dill, and olive oil.
1 tablespoon chopped fresh dill	
2 tablespoons extra-virgin olive oil	

Per serving: Calories 93 (From Fat 56); Fat 6g (Saturated 1g); Cholesterol 9mg; Sodium 759mg; Carbohydrate 2g (Dietary Fiber 1g); Protein 8g

Tip: This recipe works best with thick asparagus spears as opposed to thin ones that are more flexible.

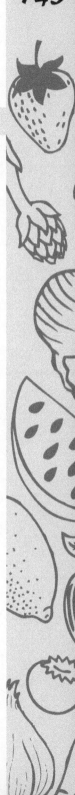

Enjoying Stuffed Starters and Wraps

Sometimes the only way to make good food even better is to combine it with yet another good food — or two. The recipes in this section take ingredients that are good standing alone — portobello mushrooms, for instance — and give them some anti-inflammatory flourish with additional ingredients.

These recipes are a treat for the distinguishing palate, a combination of spices, textures, and flavors that all blend together in an anti-inflammatory bouquet. Garlic, onions, turmeric, curry spice, and ginger are especially anti-inflammatory, and you can add them to almost any appetizer (or meal, for that matter) to boost the anti-inflammatory benefit.

A great combination to have on hand is peeled and minced fresh ginger, garlic, and some extra-virgin olive oil; these three ingredients add a pungent note to any meal and have antibacterial, antiviral, antioxidant, and anti-inflammatory properties.

Crispy Kale-Stuffed Portobello Mushrooms

Prep time: 15 min • **Cook time:** 8 min • **Yield:** 6 servings

Ingredients	Directions
6 tablespoons chopped kale 1 teaspoon wheat-free tamari sauce 2 teaspoons chopped fresh parsley 1 teaspoon chopped fresh mint ½ teaspoon garlic powder 6 portobello mushrooms Extra-virgin olive oil	*1* Preheat the oven to 350 degrees. Mix together the kale, tamari sauce, parsley, mint, and garlic powder in a small bowl. *2* Place the mushrooms with the stems up on a baking sheet brushed with olive oil. Bake them for 5 minutes. *3* Take the mushrooms out of the oven and remove the stems. Finely chop the stems and add them to the kale mixture. Mix well. *4* Place a heaping teaspoon of the kale mixture in the center of each mushroom. Bake the mushrooms for another 2 to 3 minutes. Serve hot.

Per serving: Calories 37 (From Fat 8); Fat 1g (Saturated 0g); Cholesterol 0mg; Sodium 60mg; Carbohydrate 5g (Dietary Fiber 1g); Protein 2g

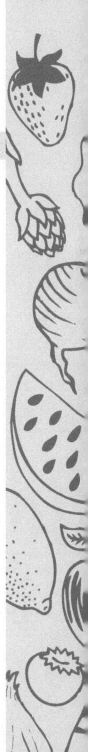

Lettuce Wraps with Brown Rice and Chickpeas

Prep time: 1 hr • **Cook time:** None • **Yield:** 4 servings

Ingredients	*Directions*
1¼ cups cooked brown rice 1 onion, chopped	*1* In a medium bowl, combine the cooked rice with the onion, parsley, mint, and chickpeas.
1½ cups chopped flat-leaf parsley 2 tablespoons chopped fresh mint	*2* In a small bowl, combine the olive oil, lemon juice, turmeric, cumin, cayenne pepper (if desired), and salt. Pour the dressing over the rice mixture and mix well.
15 ounces canned chickpeas, rinsed and drained, or 2 cups cooked chickpeas	*3* Wash, dry, and arrange the lettuce leaves on a plate. Scoop the rice mixture into the lettuce leaves and roll them up, tucking the sides inside.
6 tablespoons extra-virgin olive oil	
6 tablespoons freshly squeezed lemon juice	
1 teaspoon turmeric	
1 teaspoon cumin	
½ teaspoon ground red cayenne pepper (optional)	
1 teaspoon sea salt	
8–10 whole red lettuce leaves	

Per serving: Calories 345 (From Fat 199); Fat 22g (Saturated 3g); Cholesterol 0mg; Sodium 720mg; Carbohydrate 32g (Dietary Fiber 6g); Protein 7g

Marbled Deviled Eggs

Prep time: 20 min • **Cook time:** 5–8 min • **Yield:** 6 servings

Ingredients	*Directions*
6 eggs	*1* Boil the eggs until they're cooked, about 10 to 12 minutes. Remove the eggs from the water and crack them all around gently with the back of a spoon, leaving the shells in place.
1 teaspoon turmeric, divided	
2 tablespoons plain Greek yogurt, 0–2% fat, or nondairy cheese	
1 tablespoon Dijon mustard	*2* Add ¼ teaspoon turmeric to the boiling water. Return the eggs to the water with the turmeric, and remove the saucepan from the heat to cool.
1 tablespoon Worcestershire sauce	
⅛ teaspoon sea salt	*3* After the eggs have cooled, remove them from the water and remove the outer cracked shell.
1 tablespoon chopped fresh parsley	
1 teaspoon paprika	*4* Cut the eggs in half and scoop out the yolks into a small bowl.
	5 Smash together the egg yolks, yogurt or cheese, mustard, Worcestershire sauce, salt, and the remaining ¾ teaspoon turmeric. Scoop the mixture back into each half of the eggs.
	6 Top the eggs with parsley and sprinkle them with paprika. Chill the eggs before serving.

Note: Turmeric can stain your skin and surfaces orange or yellow, so it's best to wear plastic gloves to protect your hands and an apron to protect your clothing, and cover the preparation area with waxed paper or paper towels.

Per serving: Calories 88 (From Fat 51); Fat 6g (Saturated 2g); Cholesterol 212mg; Sodium 203mg; Carbohydrate 2g (Dietary Fiber 0g); Protein 7g

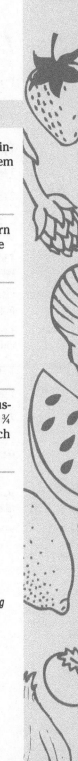

Lettuce Wraps with Spiced Turkey

Prep time: 10 min • **Cook time:** 10 min • **Yield:** 6 servings

Ingredients	Directions
1 pound ground turkey	*1* Brown the turkey in a medium skillet over medium heat. Drain any fat from the skillet.
1 large onion, chopped	
2 tablespoons minced garlic	*2* Add the chopped onion, garlic, ginger, tamari sauce, cayenne pepper, and rice wine vinegar to the browned turkey. Sauté for 5 minutes, stirring occasionally, until the onion is translucent. Add the scallions, sesame seeds, and sesame oil in the last 2 minutes of cooking.
2 teaspoons fresh minced ginger	
1 tablespoon wheat-free tamari sauce	
¼ teaspoon red cayenne pepper	
1 tablespoon rice wine vinegar	*3* Wash, dry, and arrange the lettuce leaves on a plate. Scoop the turkey mixture into the lettuce leaves. Fold the leaves over the mixture and eat like a taco.
1 scallion, chopped	
1 teaspoon sesame seeds	
2 teaspoons sesame oil	
1 head red or green leaf lettuce	

Per serving: Calories 174 (From Fat 80); Fat 9g (Saturated 2g); Cholesterol 55mg; Sodium 226mg; Carbohydrate 7g (Dietary Fiber 2g); Protein 17g

Spiced Bean Zucchini Bites

Prep time: 10 min • **Cook time:** 5 min • **Yield:** 4–6 servings

Ingredients	Directions
2 tablespoons extra-virgin olive oil, divided	**1** In a medium skillet, sauté the sliced zucchini in 1 tablespoon of the olive oil, making sure to brown the zucchini on both sides. Remove from the pan.
1 zucchini, cut into ¼-inch slices	
½ cup cooked white beans	**2** Add 1 tablespoon olive oil to the pan and then add the beans and onion. Sauté for 5 minutes. Remove from the heat, stir in the dried mint, and mix in sea salt and pepper to taste.
2 tablespoons diced red onion	
1 teaspoon dried mint	
Sea salt to taste	**3** Place the zucchini slices on a serving dish and spoon 1 teaspoon of the bean mixture on top of each slice.
Freshly ground black pepper to taste	

Per serving: Calories 101 (From Fat 63); Fat 7g (Saturated 1g); Cholesterol 0mg; Sodium 146mg; Carbohydrate 8g (Dietary Fiber 3g); Protein 3g

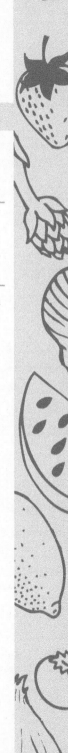

Setting Out Simple Snacks

Sometimes the best snacks are the simplest ones. You've been told since you were little that you need to eat your fruits and veggies, and we're with Mom on this one: Natural, raw vegetables are in their healthiest state because none of the nutrients have been cooked out. Dried fruit, when prepared without sugars or sulfites, provides all the necessary vitamins without added sugars.

Want something a little salty or with a crunch? Grab a handful of nuts, filled with antioxidants and protein to keep you going all day.

A pungent, anti-inflammatory appetizer from Korea that you can buy prepared at Asian food stores is called kimchee — it's made with garlic, cabbage, and anti-inflammatory herbs. Serve it as a side dish, on rice crackers, or with a main course. Check the label on store-bought kimchee to ensure it's free of additives and preservatives.

Fresh Vegetable Plate

Prep time: 10 min • **Cook time:** None • **Yield:** 10 servings

Ingredients	Directions
6 ribs organic celery, each cut in half lengthwise and then into three sticks	*1* Place cut vegetables on a plate.
16-ounce package organic baby carrots	*2* In a small bowl, whisk together the olive oil, apple cider vinegar, and salt. Drizzle the vegetables with the dressing mixture and serve.
1 bunch radishes, tops and tips removed	
1 large cucumber, peeled and sliced into ¼-inch rounds	
1 small daikon radish, sliced	
2 tablespoons extra-virgin olive oil	
2 tablespoons apple cider vinegar	
1 teaspoon sea salt	

Per serving: Calories 55 (From Fat 25); Fat 3g (Saturated 0g); Cholesterol 0mg; Sodium 288mg; Carbohydrate 7g (Dietary Fiber 2g); Protein 1g

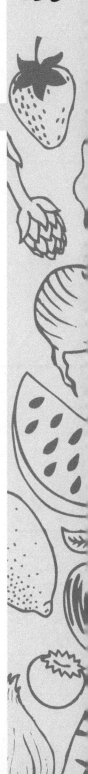

Stuffed Dates with Coconut

Prep time: 10 min • **Cook time:** None • **Yield:** 6 servings

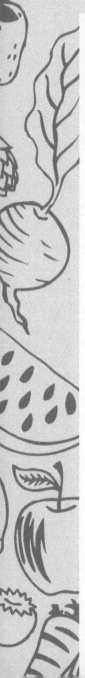

Ingredients	Directions
6 Medjool dates	*1* Slice each date down the middle and sprinkle it with coconut. Add one almond per date.
6 raw almonds	
2 tablespoons shredded coconut	

Per serving: Calories 79 (From Fat 7); Fat 1g (Saturated 0g); Cholesterol 0mg; Sodium 1mg; Carbohydrate 19g (Dietary Fiber 2g); Protein 0g

Raw Nuts and Fruit Mix

Prep time: 5 min • **Cook time:** None • **Yield:** 12 servings

Ingredients	*Directions*
8 ounces raw almonds	*1* Combine the almonds, cashews, walnuts, apple, and berries. Mix well and enjoy by the handful.
8 ounces raw cashews	
8 ounces walnuts	
½ an apple, any variety, diced	
4 ounces fresh raspberries	
4 ounces fresh blueberries	

Per serving: Calories 354 (From Fat 278); Fat 31g (Saturated 4g); Cholesterol 0mg; Sodium 9mg; Carbohydrate 15g (Dietary Fiber 5g); Protein 11g

Vary It! The fresh fruit makes this snack highly perishable. For a longer-lasting variation, try this mix with dried fruit. Use a food dehydrator to dry fresh fruit yourself, or purchase dried fruit that's free of sugars and sulfites.

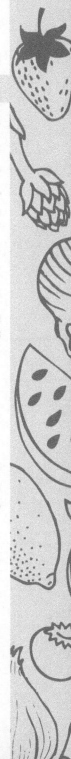

Spiced Nuts

Prep time: 10 min • **Cook time:** 30 min • **Yield:** 6 servings

Ingredients	Directions
Cooking spray	**1** Preheat the oven to 250 degrees. Spray a 9-x-13-inch baking sheet with cooking spray.
8 ounces walnuts	
8 ounces raw almonds	**2** Stir together the walnuts, almonds, five-spice powder, and salt.
2½ teaspoons five-spice powder (see the following recipe)	
¼ teaspoon sea salt	**3** In a medium bowl, whisk together the egg white and orange juice until it's light and frothy. Continue whisking as you slowly drizzle in the agave nectar.
1 large egg white	
4 teaspoons orange juice	**4** Add the spiced nuts to the egg white mixture and gently toss to coat the nuts. Spread the nuts on the baking sheet and bake for 30 minutes, or until the nuts are slightly golden. Stir the nuts around at least once during baking to avoid burning.
¼ cup agave nectar	
	5 Let the nuts cool for 5 minutes before serving.

Five-Spice Powder

½ teaspoon whole Szechuan peppercorns	**1** Use a peppermill to grind the peppercorns, cloves, and fennel seeds. Stir in the cinnamon and star anise.
½ teaspoon whole cloves	
½ teaspoon fennel seeds	
½ teaspoon ground cinnamon	
½ teaspoon powdered star anise	

Per serving: Calories 514 (From Fat 395); Fat 44g (Saturated 4g); Cholesterol 0mg; Sodium 117mg; Carbohydrate 24g (Dietary Fiber 7g); Protein 15g

Tip: If you're short on time, five-spice powder is available at most Asian food stores.

Chapter 11

Bring Out the Bowls: Soups

In This Chapter

▶ Making meatless soups

▶ Creating ethnic fare

▶ Sipping soup for the omnivore

Sometimes there's just nothing better than a bowl of soup. It doesn't have to be winter or a blustery, rainy day; soup can be a light yet filling meal that seems to hit just the right spot any time of the year.

The recipes in this chapter range from simple throw-it-in-the-blender gazpacho to more complex soups that require soaking beans overnight and working with miso or seaweed. All recipes are tailored to keep inflammation at bay, offering a hearty meal or smaller portions for a nice side.

Finding Variety in Vegetarian Soups

Vegetarian (meatless) recipes are lower in saturated fat and higher in fiber than those that contain meat. Meat is also a source of the saturated fat *arachidonic acid,* which promotes inflammation in the body in high amounts. A diet that's higher in plant sources of protein, such as beans, nuts, and seeds, can help decrease cholesterol, improve bowel function, and reduce the formation of the inflammatory mediators, such as arachidonic acid and inflammatory prostaglandins.

Combinations of soup staples — such as beans, lentils, barley, and peas — can even give you complete proteins from plant sources. And these ingredients have other benefits, too. For example, white beans contain an ingredient that has been shown to help with weight loss, and they're high in fiber and nutrients. Lentils are high in folate and iron in addition to fiber. And peas are high in the trace mineral molybdenum, which can help to detoxify sulfites, a common food additive; in other words, eating enough peas can make you less sensitive to sulfites found in wine and dried fruit.

Of course, vegetarian soups also provide a healthy serving of vegetables that have anti-inflammatory benefits on their own. Leafy vegetables, such as mustard greens, have cholesterol-lowering capabilities due to their bile-binding capacity, directing cholesterol out of the body.

The herbs and spices in soup also offer a host of anti-inflammatory benefits. For example, turmeric contains *curcumin,* a potent component that possesses antioxidant, anti-inflammatory, antibacterial, digestive-aid function, liver- and heart-protecting benefits, and anti-cancer benefits. Thyme is high in the antioxidant compounds called *flavonoids* and may help to protect the brain against aging. And rosemary and sage provide additional anti-inflammatory and antioxidant properties and a delicious taste.

Use organic soup ingredients whenever possible to minimize the addition of toxic pesticides and enhance the nutrient content of your food. Look for organic sources of spices and use them within a year to maintain their freshness and potency.

Barley and White Bean Soup

Prep time: 10 min plus overnight soak • **Cook time:** 1 hr • **Yield:** 6–8 servings

Ingredients	*Directions*
16 ounces dried cannellini beans	*1* Soak the beans in water overnight. Discard the water and rinse the beans.
2 tablespoons extra-virgin olive oil	*2* Warm the olive oil in a large stock pot over medium-low heat. Sauté the onion and garlic until the onions are translucent, about 5 minutes.
1 white onion, diced	
2 cloves garlic, minced	
2 cups organic vegetable broth or chicken broth	*3* Add the broth, water, barley or rice, carrots and soaked beans to the saucepan. Bring the soup to a boil over high heat.
9 cups water	
½ cup barley or brown rice	*4* Lower the heat to medium, add the sage and rosemary, and simmer the soup for about 1 hour, or until the beans and barley or rice are cooked through. Add more water as needed for desired thickness. Season the soup to taste with salt and pepper.
2 large carrots, peeled and cut into ¼-inch slices	
1 tablespoon dried sage	
2 tablespoons dried rosemary	
Sea salt to taste	
Freshly ground black pepper to taste	

Per serving: Calories 385 (From Fat 61); Fat 7g (Saturated 1g); Cholesterol 2mg; Sodium 451mg; Carbohydrate 63g (Dietary Fiber 15g); Protein 20g

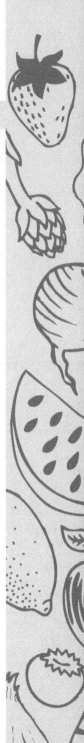

Lentil and Greens Soup

Prep time: 10 min • **Cook time:** 40–50 min • **Yield:** 6–8 servings

Ingredients	*Directions*
2 tablespoons extra-virgin olive oil	*1* Warm the olive oil in a large stock pot over medium-low heat. Sauté the onions and garlic until the onions are translucent, about 5 minutes.
1 onion, diced	
2 cloves garlic, minced	
6 cups organic vegetable broth or chicken broth	*2* Add the broth, water, coriander, cumin, turmeric, and rinsed lentils. Bring to a boil over high heat; then reduce the heat and simmer for 20 to 40 minutes or until the lentils are soft. Add the mustard greens in the last 5 minutes of cooking.
2 cups water	
1 teaspoon ground coriander seed	
1 teaspoon ground cumin seed	*3* Season the soup to taste with salt and pepper. Add the lemon juice and fresh parsley to the soup just before serving.
½ teaspoon turmeric	
1 pound brown or green lentils, rinsed	
½ cup mustard greens, chopped	
Juice of 2 lemons	
¼ cup fresh parsley	
Sea salt to taste	
Freshly ground black pepper to taste	

Per serving: Calories 333 (From Fat 55); Fat 6g (Saturated 1g); Cholesterol 0mg; Sodium 468mg; Carbohydrate 53g (Dietary Fiber 19g); Protein 21g

Northern Bean Soup

Prep time: 10 min plus overnight soak • **Cook time:** 1–2 hrs • **Yield:** 6 servings

Ingredients	*Directions*
1 pound dry great Northern beans 1 piece dried Kombu seaweed	*1* Soak the beans in water overnight with the piece of seaweed. Discard the water and seaweed, and rinse the beans.
4 cups organic vegetable broth or chicken broth 4 cups water ½ cup chopped carrots ½ cup chopped celery 1 large leek, washed well and chopped 1 tablespoon dried thyme	*2* Combine the beans, broth, water, carrots, celery, leek, and dried thyme in a large stock pot. Bring the soup to a boil over high heat; then reduce the heat and simmer for 90 minutes or until the beans are cooked.
Sea salt to taste Freshly ground black pepper to taste	*3* Season the soup to taste with salt and pepper.

Tip: Soaking the beans overnight with a piece of dried Kombu seaweed helps decrease the amount of gas formed from eating beans. The seaweed may be found in some Asian markets as well as on various websites, including www.amazon.com and www.foodservice direct.com.

Per serving: Calories 252 (From Fat 12); Fat 1g (Saturated 0g); Cholesterol 0mg; Sodium 422mg; Carbohydrate 46g (Dietary Fiber 15g); Protein 17g

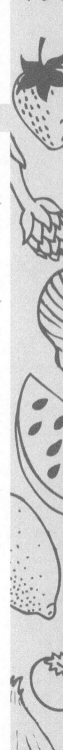

Butternut Squash, Sweet Potato, and White Bean Stew

Prep time: 10 min, plus overnight soak • **Cook time:** 1 hr • **Yield:** 6–8 servings

Ingredients	*Directions*
1 pound dried cannellini beans	*1* Soak the beans in water overnight. Discard the water and rinse the beans.
32 ounces organic vegetable broth or chicken broth	*2* Bring the broth and water to a boil in a large stock pot.
2 cups water	
2 cloves garlic, minced	*3* Add the white beans, garlic, onion, ginger, lemon zest, and rosemary to the broth and lower the heat to a simmer. Cook for 40 minutes or until the beans soften.
1 small sweet onion, chopped	
1 tablespoon ground ginger	
1 tablespoon lemon zest	*4* Add the sweet potatoes and butternut squash and cook for another 20 minutes or until the sweet potatoes are soft and easily pierced with a fork.
1 tablespoon crushed dried rosemary	
2 sweet potatoes, peeled and cut into 1-inch pieces	
1 butternut squash, peeled, and cut into 1-inch pieces	
Sea salt to taste	

Per serving: Calories 347 (From Fat 9); Fat 1g (Saturated 0g); Cholesterol 0mg; Sodium 476mg; Carbohydrate 68g (Dietary Fiber 15g); Protein 20g

Yellow Split Pea Soup

Prep time: 10 min • **Cook time:** 1 hr • **Yield:** 6 servings

Ingredients	Directions
2 tablespoons extra-virgin olive oil	*1* Warm the olive oil in a large stock pot over medium-low heat, and sauté the onions until they're translucent, about 5 minutes.
2 medium onions, diced	
6 cups organic vegetable broth or chicken broth	*2* Add the broth, split peas, carrots, potatoes, and marjoram to the onion. Bring the soup to a boil over high heat, and then reduce the heat to simmer for up to 1 hour or until the potatoes are cooked through and the soup is a desired thickness. Season the soup to taste with salt and pepper.
1 pound dried yellow split peas	
½ cup diced carrots	
1 large potato, peeled and diced	
2 teaspoons dried marjoram	
Sea salt to taste	
Freshly ground black pepper to taste	

Per serving: Calories 334 (From Fat 53); Fat 6g (Saturated 1g); Cholesterol 0mg; Sodium 549mg; Carbohydrate 56g (Dietary Fiber 19g); Protein 18g

Tip: Test the doneness of the diced potatoes by spearing a couple with a fork. If they slide off the fork easily, they're done.

Note: White potatoes are part of the nightshade family and are optional in this recipe. For something different, try parsnips or sweet potatoes.

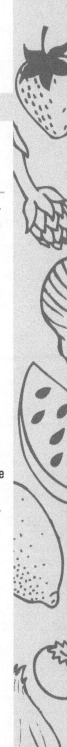

Cabbage Soup

Prep time: 10 min • **Cook time:** 30–45 min • **Yield:** 4 servings

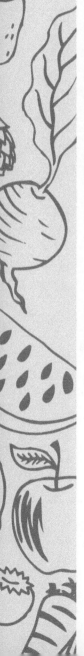

Ingredients	*Directions*
½ head of green cabbage, about 4 cups chopped	*1* Chop the cabbage, celery, carrots, and onions. Put them in a large stock pot with the sliced mushrooms.
3 stalks celery	
2 carrots	*2* Add the vegetable broth and water and bring the mixture to a boil over high heat. Reduce the heat, add the chopped rosemary and thyme, and simmer the soup for 30 minutes or until the carrots and cabbage are soft.
1 large onion	
1 cup sliced crimini mushrooms	
2 cups organic vegetable broth	
3 cups water	*3* Add the Swiss chard and simmer the soup for 5 minutes or until the Swiss chard is soft. Season the soup to taste with salt and pepper.
1 tablespoon dried rosemary	
1 tablespoon dried thyme	
1 bunch Swiss chard, chopped	
Sea salt to taste	
Freshly ground black pepper to taste	

Per serving: Calories 90 (From Fat 5); Fat 1g (Saturated 0g); Cholesterol 0mg; Sodium 611mg; Carbohydrate 20g (Dietary Fiber 5g); Protein 4g

Ginger Butternut Squash Soup

Prep time: 10 min • **Cook time:** 30 min • **Yield:** 6 servings

Ingredients	Directions
2 tablespoons extra-virgin olive oil	*1* Warm the olive oil in a large stock pot over medium-low heat, and sauté the onions until they're translucent, about 5 minutes.
1 medium onion, chopped	
6 cups organic vegetable broth or chicken broth	*2* Add the broth, butternut squash, and ginger to the onion and bring the soup to a boil over high heat. Reduce the heat, cover, and simmer the soup for 20 minutes or until the squash is soft.
1 butternut squash, peeled and cubed	
1-inch piece of fresh ginger, minced	*3* Let the soup cool for a few minutes before transferring it to a blender or food processor. Blend or process the soup until it's smooth.
½ cup plain Greek yogurt, 0–2% fat (optional)	
2 tablespoons ground coriander seed	*4* Serve each bowl with a tablespoon of Greek yogurt (if desired) and a sprinkling of ground coriander.

Per serving: Calories 115 (From Fat 49); Fat 5g (Saturated 1g); Cholesterol 0mg; Sodium 464mg; Carbohydrate 16g (Dietary Fiber 4g); Protein 2g

Tip: To minimize cleanup, skip the blender or food processer and use an immersion blender in Step 3.

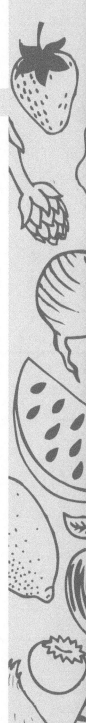

Pumpkin Soup with Pine Nuts

Prep time: 10 min • **Cook time:** 30 min • **Yield:** 8 servings

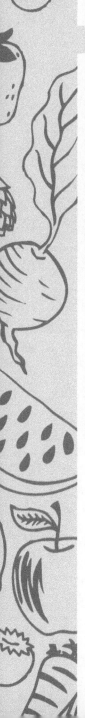

Ingredients	Directions
8 cups organic vegetable broth or chicken broth	*1* Put the broth in a large stock pot and bring to a boil over high heat.
1 medium sugar pumpkin, seeded, peeled, and chopped	
1 large sweet onion, chopped	*2* Add the pumpkin, onion, nutmeg, allspice, and 1 teaspoon cinnamon to the broth. Reduce the heat and simmer the soup until the pumpkin is cooked, approximately 20 to 30 minutes. Add the honey in the last 5 minutes of cooking.
¼ teaspoon ground nutmeg	
¼ teaspoon allspice	
2 teaspoons cinnamon, divided	
¼ teaspoon raw, unprocessed honey	*3* Let the soup cool for a few minutes before transferring it to a blender or food processor. Blend or process the soup until it's smooth.
½ cup plain Greek yogurt, 0–2% fat (optional)	*4* Serve each bowl with a tablespoon of Greek yogurt (if desired), ½ tablespoon pine nuts, and a sprinkling of the remaining cinnamon.
4 tablespoons pine nuts	

Per serving: Calories 75 (From Fat 25); Fat 3g (Saturated 0g); Cholesterol 0mg; Sodium 461mg; Carbohydrate 11g (Dietary Fiber 2g); Protein 3g

Tip: If you can't find a sugar pumpkin or if you're short on time, use 8 ounces of canned organic pumpkin puree instead of the sugar pumpkin. Simmer the soup until the onion is cooked, and skip Step 3 (pureeing the soup until smooth).

Zucchini Harvest Soup

Prep time: 10 min • **Cook time:** 35–40 min • **Yield:** 8 servings

Ingredients	Directions
3 tablespoons extra-virgin olive oil	**1** Warm the olive oil in a large stock pot over medium heat. Sauté the zucchini and garlic until they're soft, about 5 minutes.
4 cups chopped zucchini	
1 clove garlic, minced	**2** Put the onion, parsley, and water in a food processor. Blend them until smooth.
1 sweet onion, roughly chopped	
½ cup fresh parsley	**3** To the zucchini and garlic, add the vegetable broth and onion mixture. Bring the soup to a boil over high heat; then reduce the heat and simmer for 30 minutes.
1 cup water	
6 cups organic vegetable broth	
2 teaspoons dried tarragon	**4** Stir in the tarragon and let the soup cool for a few minutes. Serve each bowl of soup with a lemon wedge.
1 lemon, cut into wedges	

Per serving: Calories 88 (From Fat 50); Fat 6g (Saturated 1g); Cholesterol 0mg; Sodium 350mg; Carbohydrate 8g (Dietary Fiber 2g); Protein 2g

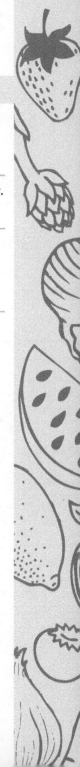

Soups with an Asian Twist

The soups in this section contain immune-stimulating ingredients such as shiitake mushrooms, garlic, ginger, and mustard. Ginger, which is common in Asian cooking, is a rhizome (similar to a root) that has a pungent taste and offers many health benefits. Researchers have studied ginger extensively for its antioxidant, anti-inflammatory, antibacterial, and antiviral benefits, and it's been used for thousands of years to aid digestion and reduce the occurrence of spasms in the colon. Ginger is also very helpful for relieving nausea.

Miso, which has been part of Japanese cooking since the sixth or seventh century, is a soybean paste made by fermenting rice, barley, or soy with salt and *Aspergillus oryzae,* a fungus long used in miso and soy sauce. Miso is high in protein, vitamins, minerals, and probiotics. It comes in different variations, such as white, red, and mixed miso. The lighter-colored miso is less salty, while the darker colors are saltier and have a bolder flavor.

Types of miso vary based on their ingredients, but they all have equal health benefits. All have a soybean base, but many have additional ingredients: For example, *kome miso* is also made with white rice; *mugi miso* is made from barley; *soba miso* is made from buckwheat; *genmai miso* is made with brown rice; and *natto miso* is made with ginger. *Hatcho miso* has no other ingredients.

Though all the Asian ingredients in the following recipes may be found in Asian markets, more and more supermarkets are carrying ingredients for ethnic cooking, as well.

Don't boil miso paste. Heat kills its nutrients. Rather, boil water or broth first and add miso paste at the end of the cooking time.

Miso Soup with Tofu and Kale

Prep time: 10 min • **Cook time:** 15 min • **Yield:** 4 servings

Ingredients	*Directions*
6 cups water	*1* Bring the water to a boil in a large stock pot over high heat. Add the shiitake mushrooms, enoki mushrooms, tofu, kale, seaweed, and radish. Reduce the heat and simmer for 10 minutes.
½ cup sliced shiitake mushrooms	
¼ cup chopped enoki mushrooms	*2* Turn off the heat and add the scallions to the soup. Remove the pot from the heat and dissolve the miso paste in the soup. Serve immediately.
1 cup cubed firm tofu	
¼ cup chopped kale	
1 piece Nori seaweed, chopped	
2-inch piece of daikon (white) radish, chopped	
1 scallion, chopped	
2 tablespoons miso paste	

Per serving: Calories 115 (From Fat 50); Fat 6g (Saturated 1g); Cholesterol 0mg; Sodium 325mg; Carbohydrate 8g (Dietary Fiber 2g); Protein 11g

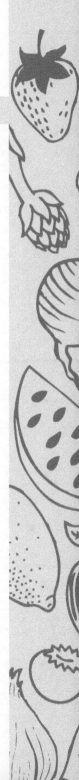

Miso Soup with Noodles

Prep time: 5 min • **Cook time:** 10 min • **Yield:** 4 servings

Ingredients	Directions
1 tablespoon extra-virgin olive oil	*1* Warm the olive oil in a large stock pot over medium-low heat. Add the garlic, ginger, and mustard seeds. Cook for about 30 seconds.
2 cloves garlic, minced	
1 tablespoon minced fresh ginger	*2* Add the mushrooms to the pot and continue to cook for 3 to 5 minutes or until you hear the mustard seeds pop.
1 tablespoon mustard seeds	
1 cup sliced shiitake mushrooms	*3* Add the water to the pot and bring the soup to a boil over high heat.
6 cups water	
8 ounces soba or rice noodles	*4* Add the noodles and seaweed and boil for 3 minutes. Stir in the scallions and remove the soup from the heat.
1 piece Nori seaweed, chopped	
2 scallions, chopped	*5* Dissolve the miso paste in the soup and serve.
2 tablespoons miso paste	

Per serving: Calories 293 (From Fat 44); Fat 5g (Saturated 1g); Cholesterol 0mg; Sodium 443mg; Carbohydrate 55g (Dietary Fiber 4g); Protein 13g

Hearty Chicken Soup

If you're an omnivore rather than a vegetarian, you'll appreciate the down-home goodness of the chicken soup in this section, which is chock full of anti-inflammatory benefits.

Use organic meat to minimize exposure to hormones, toxins, and antibiotics.

One ingredient we like for anti-inflammation cooking is kale because it's high in flavonoids (such as quercetin), which have antioxidant and anti-inflammatory benefits and help your body detoxify. Figure 11-1 shows you how to chop kale for this recipe and others.

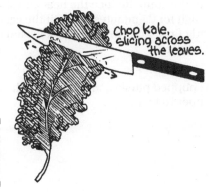

Figure 11-1:
Chopping
kale.

Chicken Soup with Kale

Prep time: 10 min • **Cook time:** 30 min • **Yield:** 8 servings

Ingredients	Directions
2 tablespoons extra-virgin olive oil	*1* Warm the olive oil in a large stock pot over medium-low heat. Sauté the onions, garlic, and leek for 5 minutes. Add the broth and water to the pot, and bring the soup to a boil over high heat.
1 onion, diced	
2 cloves garlic, minced	
1 large leek, washed well and chopped	
3 cups organic chicken broth	*2* Add the carrots, celery, turnip, rice, and cooked chicken to the soup. Reduce the heat and simmer the soup on high for 25 minutes, or until the carrots are still slightly firm. Add the chopped kale and cook for 5 minutes longer.
3 cups water	
3 large carrots, peeled and diced	
2 stalks celery, diced	*3* Add the chopped parsley, and season with salt and black pepper to taste.
1 turnip, peeled and diced	
½ cup Arborio rice	
1 pound cooked chicken breast, chopped	
1 cup chopped kale	
¼ cup chopped fresh parsley	
Sea salt to taste	
Freshly ground black pepper to taste	

Per serving: Calories 235 (From Fat 72); Fat 8g (Saturated 2g); Cholesterol 51mg; Sodium 331mg; Carbohydrate 21g (Dietary Fiber 3g); Protein 19g

Tip: Make chicken soup with leftovers from a chicken dinner.

Chapter 12

Keeping It Light: Salads

In This Chapter

▶ Working with various greens and light dressings

▶ Adding meat or seafood

▶ Serving bean-based salads

Salads made from a head of lettuce and a few extra veggies are for beginners. We don't argue that sometimes a basic salad provides a tasty, fresh addition to a meal, but we want you to explore the wide world of salads — both side salads and heartier entree-types — and the variety of anti-inflammatory ingredients that you can experiment with. For example, toss in a little protein in the form of legumes or seafood as well as a mixture of vegetables, and you have a dish that not only is appealing and appetizing but also fits in with your anti-inflammatory diet. In this chapter, we use a mixture of bitter greens, spinach, and red lettuce in a variety of dishes.

Portion size is important to keep in mind with salad as well as other components of your meal. Many people think that because they're eating a salad that contains lots of healthy ingredients, they can eat as much as they want. Wrong! Too much of anything is never a good thing, and salads are no exception. There are definite daily limits on some ingredients — like nuts, for example — that shouldn't be ignored (consult the anti-inflammatory food pyramid in Chapter 4), and you need to be conscientious about any dressing you put on your salad as well.

How much dressing is appropriate? We've all had bites of salad that seemed to have more dressing than lettuce. Rather than douse your salad in dressing, control your portion size by putting your dressing on the side and dipping your fork into it for each bite of lettuce.

Starring Greens and Other Veggies

There's good reason the base color of any good salad is green. You probably know the benefits of leafy greens when it comes to weight management, as most are typically pretty low in calories. But did you know that greens are also rich in dietary fiber, folic acid, vitamin C, potassium, and magnesium, as well as low in fat? This winning combination adds up to a reduced risk of heart disease and cancer. Because of their high magnesium levels, leafy greens can also help people with diabetes.

When you've created the mighty green base of your salad — whether it comes from spinach, kale, romaine, or arugula — be sure to add the right toppers. Cruciferous veggies like broccoli, cauliflower, and cabbage are bursting with anti-aging and cancer-fighting phytonutrients as well as calcium, iron, and folic acid. The vitamin K and folate in carrots help fight cancer and improve eyesight. And certain "root" foods such as leeks, garlic, onions, and shallots contain high levels of antibiotic properties.

Growing your own greens

Growing your own lettuce and greens is an easy and convenient way to make sure you have the fresh greens on hand for an anti-inflammatory salad anytime you want. Greens can be grown in containers or in the ground; they need very little space and grow quickly. Not sure what kinds of greens to start with? There's a variety of seeds available for all climates and growing conditions, so start with a mixture. Try some greens that you're already familiar with, like spinach, romaine, and arugula, but don't be afraid to mix in some new-to-you varieties as well.

After you've decided what to plant, you need to figure out how to plant them: Do you want container plants that you can line your patio or deck with, or do you have an established garden already in the ground? Here are some tips on both methods:

✔ **Containers:** Start with good organic potting soil in the container, and moisten the soil thoroughly. Because lettuce seeds are small and don't need much depth, you can simply sprinkle the seeds on top of the soil and then cover with about ¼ inch of new soil. To moisten the topsoil, use a spray bottle or mister to keep the seeds from floating to the top.

✔ **Grounded:** Many experts recommend planting lettuce and greens in direct sun about two weeks before the projected last frost in your area. Seeds should be planted about ¼ to ½ inch below the surface and about 2 inches apart, covered with fresh soil. Once the seedlings start to appear, thin the plants (by removing some selectively) so they're about 12 inches apart. Be sure to keep the soil moist as the plants grow; letting them be dry for too long may give them a bitter taste come harvest time.

Spinach Salad with Balsamic Vinaigrette

Prep time: 10 min • **Cook time:** None • **Yield:** 2 servings

Ingredients	Directions
6 tablespoons extra-virgin olive oil	*1* Make a vinaigrette by whisking together the olive oil, balsamic vinegar, white wine vinegar, mint, and sea salt.
1 teaspoon balsamic vinegar	
3 tablespoons white wine vinegar	*2* Arrange the spinach on two plates. Top it with black raspberries, apple slices, and the slivered almonds. Sprinkle goat cheese on top (if desired).
½ teaspoon chopped fresh mint or ¼ teaspoon dried mint	
Sea salt to taste	*3* Drizzle the salad with the vinaigrette or serve the dressing on the side.
2 cups fresh baby spinach	
¼ cup black raspberries	
1 tart apple, thinly sliced	
2 tablespoons slivered almonds	
2 tablespoons crumbled goat cheese (optional)	

Per serving: Calories 496 (From Fat 417); Fat 46g (Saturated 7g); Cholesterol 6mg; Sodium 365mg; Carbohydrate 20g (Dietary Fiber 4g); Protein 4g

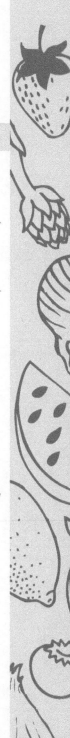

Broccoli Salad

Prep time: 10 min • **Cook time:** 5–10 min • **Yield:** 2 servings

Ingredients	Directions
¼ cup water	**1** Lightly steam the broccoli crowns in a pan with ¼ cup of water over medium heat, about 5 to 7 minutes. (A steamer basket is recommended but isn't necessary.) Put the chopped endive and walnuts in a medium bowl.
3 cups chopped broccoli crowns	
½ cup chopped endive	
½ cup walnuts	**2** Strain the broccoli and immediately combine it with the endive and walnuts.
1 tablespoon extra-virgin olive oil	
1 teaspoon red pepper flakes, or to taste	**3** Toss the broccoli mix with olive oil and red pepper flakes.

Per serving: Calories 263 (From Fat 214); Fat 24g (Saturated 3g); Cholesterol 0mg; Sodium 30mg; Carbohydrate 11g (Dietary Fiber 6g); Protein 7g

Crunchy Vegetable Salad with Beets and Eggs

Prep time: 20 min • **Cook time:** None • **Yield:** 2 servings

Ingredients	*Directions*
2 cups mesclun greens	*1* Line two plates with the mesclun greens.
1 raw yellow beet, peeled and grated	*2* Place the grated beet in a small bowl with olive oil and white wine vinegar. Add the radish, chives, and 1 tablespoon parsley to the grated beets and mix gently. Spoon the beet mixture onto the greens.
1 teaspoon olive oil	
1 teaspoon white wine vinegar	
1 medium radish, diced	*3* Peel the hard-boiled eggs, slice them in half, and serve the halves on the side of the salad.
2 tablespoons chopped fresh chives	
2 tablespoons chopped fresh parsley, divided	*4* Sprinkle the salad with the remaining parsley, salt, and black pepper to taste.
2 eggs, hard-boiled	
Sea salt to taste	
Freshly ground black pepper to taste	

Per serving: Calories 129 (From Fat 70); Fat 8g (Saturated 2g); Cholesterol 212mg; Sodium 400mg; Carbohydrate 7g (Dietary Fiber 3g); Protein 8g

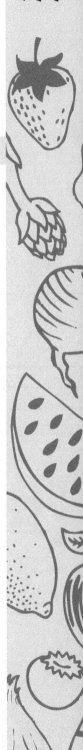

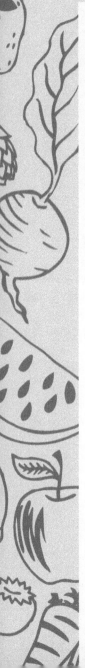

Greek Cucumber Salad with Rosemary

Prep time: 10 min plus refrigerating time • **Cook time:** None • **Yield:** 2 servings

Ingredients	*Directions*
2 large cucumbers, sliced	*1* Combine the cucumber, red onions, feta cheese (if desired), and olives.
1 small red onion, sliced	
1 cup crumbled feta cheese (optional)	*2* Whisk together the olive oil, balsamic vinegar, and rosemary. Add the dressing to the cucumber mixture and toss gently to combine. Refrigerate 1 to 2 hours for the flavors to marry before serving.
¼ cup Kalamata olives	
8 tablespoons extra-virgin olive oil	
3 tablespoons balsamic vinegar	
1 teaspoon dried rosemary	

Per serving: Calories 583 (From Fat 527); Fat 59g (Saturated 8g); Cholesterol 0mg; Sodium 257mg; Carbohydrate 15g (Dietary Fiber 3g); Protein 3g

Arugula Salad with Chickpeas and Grapes

Prep time: 5 min • **Cook time:** None • **Yield:** 2 servings

Ingredients	Directions
2 cups chopped arugula	**1** Combine the arugula and celery. Add the chickpeas, grapes, and walnuts and toss to combine.
1 large celery stalk, chopped	
½ cup cooked chickpeas	**2** Whisk together the olive oil and red wine vinegar. Place the salad on two plates, and drizzle with the dressing or serve the dressing on the side.
¼ cup halved red grapes	
1 tablespoon chopped walnuts	
2 tablespoons extra-virgin olive oil	
1 tablespoon red wine vinegar	

Per serving: Calories 233 (From Fat 152); Fat 17g (Saturated 2g); Cholesterol 0mg; Sodium 34mg; Carbohydrate 18g (Dietary Fiber 4g); Protein 5g

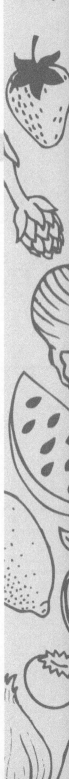

Bitter Greens Salad

Prep time: 10 min • **Cook time:** None • **Yield:** 2 servings

Ingredients	Directions
½ cup dandelion leaves	**1** Toss together the dandelion greens, mustard greens, and red lettuce. Place the salad on two plates and top with avocado slices.
½ cup chopped mustard greens	
1 cup chopped red lettuce	
1 large avocado, peeled, pitted, and sliced	**2** Whisk together the olive oil, raspberry vinegar, and chopped parsley. Drizzle the dressing over the greens or serve on the side. Sprinkle the salads with salt and black pepper to taste.
6 tablespoons extra-virgin olive oil	
2 tablespoons raspberry vinegar	
1 tablespoon chopped fresh parsley	
Sea salt to taste	
Freshly ground black pepper to taste	

Per serving: Calories 547 (From Fat 488); Fat 54g (Saturated 8g); Cholesterol 0mg; Sodium 312mg; Carbohydrate 17g (Dietary Fiber 9g); Protein 4g

Tip: This recipe calls for dandelion leaves, but you shouldn't just venture into your yard and harvest your own. For cooking and salads, the leaves are picked before the yellow flowers develop. You can find dandelion leaves in most organic markets; dried varieties are available on several websites, such as www.amazon.com and www.iHerb.com.

Making a Meal of Salads with Meat or Seafood

Your salad doesn't always have to be the sidekick to your meal. Add just a few hearty ingredients — think meat or seafood and maybe a few heavier veggies — and that little salad that used to sit on the sidelines is now featured center stage.

Salads can and often do make hearty main courses (or only courses) and provide all the anti-inflammatory benefits of many of their more traditional main meal counterparts when you add protein like meat and seafood.

Arugula Salad with Chicken

Prep time: 1 hr, 10 min • **Cook time:** 10–15 min • **Yield:** 2 servings

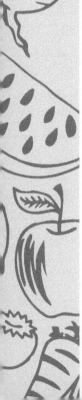

Ingredients	*Directions*
8 ounces raw chicken, cut into 1-inch strips	*1* In a plastic zip-top bag, combine the chicken strips with 2 tablespoons of the olive oil, the lemon juice, and the salt and pepper. Put the bag in the refrigerator to marinate for at least 1 hour, jostling the chicken in the bag a couple of times as it marinates to ensure full coverage.
6 tablespoons extra-virgin olive oil, divided	
Juice of 1 lemon	
Dash of sea salt	
Dash of freshly ground black pepper	*2* Adjust the oven rack so the food will be about four inches from the upper heating element. Turn on the broiler. Lay the marinated chicken strips on a baking pan and broil for 3 to 4 minutes on each side.
2 cups arugula	
2 tablespoons pistachio nuts	*3* Divide the arugula onto two plates. Top with the chicken strips, pistachios, and Gruyère cheese (if desired).
¼ cup thinly sliced Gruyère cheese (optional)	
2 tablespoons balsamic vinegar	*4* Whisk together the remaining 4 tablespoons olive oil, balsamic vinegar, and salt and pepper to taste. Pour the dressing over the salads or serve the dressing on the side.

Per serving: Calories 484 (From Fat 362); Fat 40g (Saturated 6g); Cholesterol 72mg; Sodium 399mg; Carbohydrate 6g (Dietary Fiber 1g); Protein 26g

New Cobb Salad

Prep time: 10 min • **Cook time:** None • **Yield:** 2 servings

Ingredients	*Directions*
½ cup chopped broccoli crowns	*1* Arrange the broccoli, mushrooms, turkey, and avocado in layers on two plates. Top with the sliced almonds.
½ cup chopped mushrooms	
1 cup cooked, cubed turkey breast	*2* Whisk together the olive oil, garlic, horseradish, Dijon mustard, and red wine vinegar. Drizzle the dressing on the salads or serve the dressing on the side.
1 large avocado, peeled, pitted, and sliced	
¼ cup sliced almonds	
6 tablespoons extra-virgin olive oil	
1 clove garlic, crushed	
1 tablespoon horseradish	
2 tablespoons Dijon mustard	
2 tablespoons red wine vinegar	

Per serving: Calories 732 (From Fat 558); Fat 62g (Saturated 9g); Cholesterol 59mg; Sodium 430mg; Carbohydrate 22g (Dietary Fiber 10g); Protein 29g

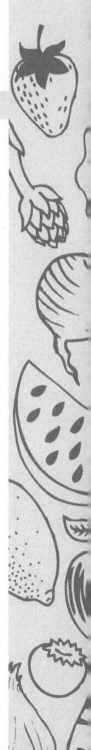

Green Salad with Spicy Shrimp

Prep time: 10 min • **Cook time:** None • **Yield:** 4 servings

Ingredients	*Directions*
4 cups mesclun greens	*1* Arrange the greens on four plates.
6 tablespoons extra-virgin olive oil	*2* Whisk together the olive oil, lemon juice, dill, and chili sauce. Toss the shrimp with the olive-oil mixture.
Juice of 2 lemons	
2 tablespoons fresh dill weed	
1 teaspoon chili sauce	*3* Top the greens with the shrimp, dividing it among the four plates. Top the salads with cilantro and salt to taste.
1 pound medium peeled, cooked shrimp	
¼ cup fresh chopped cilantro	
Sea salt to taste	

Per serving: Calories 308 (From Fat 195); Fat 22g (Saturated 3g); Cholesterol 221mg; Sodium 453mg; Carbohydrate 4g (Dietary Fiber 1g); Protein 25g

Salmon and Pear Salad

Prep time: 10 min • **Cook time:** None • **Yield:** 4 servings

Ingredients	Directions
1 head red lettuce, chopped	*1* Arrange the lettuce on four plates. Top the lettuce with the salmon, walnuts, scallions, pears, and Gorgonzola cheese (if desired).
1 pound broiled wild salmon	
¼ cup chopped walnuts	
2 scallions, chopped	*2* Whisk together the lemon juice, olive oil, and white wine vinegar. Pour the dressing over the salads or serve the dressing on the side. Season with black pepper to taste.
1 small pear, thinly sliced	
½ cup Gorgonzola cheese (optional)	
Juice of 1 lemon	
6 tablespoons extra-virgin olive oil	
2 tablespoons white wine vinegar	
Freshly ground black pepper to taste	

Per serving: Calories 468 (From Fat 306); Fat 34g (Saturated 5g); Cholesterol 81mg; Sodium 78mg; Carbohydrate 11g (Dietary Fiber 3g); Protein 32g

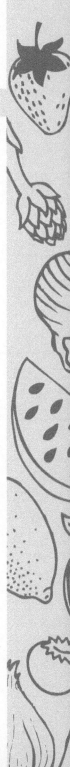

Pomegranate, Walnut, and Tuna Salad

Prep time: 10 min • **Cook time:** None • **Yield:** 1 serving

Ingredients	*Directions*
1 cup fresh baby spinach	*1* Place the spinach on a salad plate.
2 teaspoons extra-virgin olive oil	
1 teaspoon apple cider vinegar	*2* Whisk together the olive oil and cider vinegar. Mix in the tuna and feta cheese (if desired). Spoon the tuna mixture on top of the spinach.
5 ounces canned albacore tuna in water, drained	
¼ cup crumbled feta cheese (optional)	*3* Top the salad with the walnuts and pomegranate seeds.
2 tablespoons chopped walnuts	
2 tablespoons fresh pomegranate seeds	

Per serving: Calories 378 (From Fat 204); Fat 23g (Saturated 3g); Cholesterol 0mg; Sodium 394mg; Carbohydrate 8g (Dietary Fiber 2g); Protein 36g

Tip: To easily and more cleanly remove the seeds from a pomegranate, cut the crown from the fruit and quarter the flesh, being careful not to puncture the seeds. Immerse the pomegranate quarters in a bowl of water and carefully separate the pomegranate at the perforations. With your hands still in the water, separate the seeds from the membrane and the flesh.

Mackerel and Cucumber Salad

Prep time: 10 min • **Cook time:** None • **Yield:** 2 servings

Ingredients	Directions
1 medium cucumber 1 small fennel bulb	*1* Chop the cucumber and the white portion of the fennel. Drain the mackerel and reserve the olive oil.
8 ounces canned mackerel packed in olive oil ¼ cup olives	*2* Combine the cucumber and fennel with the mackerel and olives. Place the salad on two plates and top with parsley.
2 tablespoons fresh chopped parsley Juice of 1 lemon	*3* Whisk together the reserved olive oil from the mackerel and the lemon juice. Drizzle the dressing on top of the salads or serve the dressing on the side.

Per serving: Calories 448 (From Fat 241); Fat 27g (Saturated 6g); Cholesterol 69mg; Sodium 956mg; Carbohydrate 25g (Dietary Fiber 9g); Protein 29g

Note: Some mackerel can contain high levels of metals. A good choice is Portuguese mackerel, or you can substitute salmon for mackerel in this recipe.

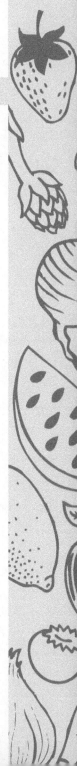

Fixing Bean Salads

If you love beans, you know which types you prefer and how to cook them. But if beans aren't already a staple in your diet, you may be wondering which of the many bean varieties out there are best for your anti-inflammatory diet, and you may not be sure of whether you should use canned beans or dried.

Truth is, there's very little nutritional difference between dried and canned beans — aside from their sodium levels. Both varieties are rich in protein and fiber and offer many essential vitamins and nutrients. According to the United States Department of Agriculture, one cup of canned navy beans has 1174 mg of sodium, while one cup of prepared dried navy beans has zero sodium. It's an important difference if you're watching your salt intake, which is a concern if you have obesity issues, heart disease, or diabetes. Draining and rinsing the canned beans is one good way to reduce sodium levels.

Probably the biggest reason many people choose canned beans over the dried variety, however, has to do with convenience. Most dried beans have to soak for hours before being cooked, while canned beans can be used right out of the can.

Make using dried beans easier by soaking more than you need for a particular recipe. Freeze what you don't need right away for use later. Or plan to soak beans overnight so they're ready when you are.

Red Bean Salad

Prep time: 5 min • **Cook time:** None • **Yield:** 6–8 servings

Ingredients	*Directions*
1 red bell pepper, cored, seeded, and chopped	*1* Combine the red bell pepper, green bell pepper, red onion, and tomato. Add the kidney beans, pinto beans, chile pepper, cilantro, lime juice, and olive oil. Gently mix.
1 green bell pepper, cored, seeded, and chopped	
1 red onion, chopped	*2* Season to taste with sea salt.
1 large tomato, chopped	
15 ounces canned red kidney beans, rinsed and drained	
15 ounces canned pinto beans, rinsed and drained	
2 tablespoons diced serrano chile peppers	
¼ cup chopped cilantro	
Juice of 2 limes	
¼ cup extra-virgin olive oil	
Sea salt to taste	

Per serving: Calories 191 (From Fat 83); Fat 9g (Saturated 1g); Cholesterol 0mg; Sodium 269mg; Carbohydrate 22g (Dietary Fiber 6g); Protein 6g

Note: This recipe contains several members of the nightshade family, including peppers and tomatoes, and therefore isn't recommended if you have a sensitivity to nightshades.

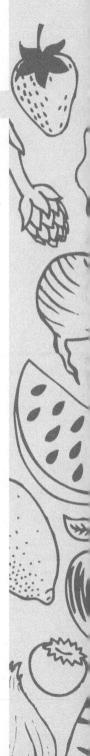

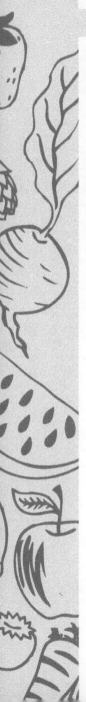

White Bean Salad

Prep time: 5 min plus refrigerating time • **Cook time:** None • **Yield:** 4 servings

Ingredients	*Directions*
4 tablespoons extra-virgin olive oil	*1* Whisk together the olive oil, vinegar, shallot, and parsley. Mix in the beans and watercress.
2 tablespoons white wine vinegar	
1 shallot, diced	*2* Sprinkle the salads with rosemary and thyme. Refrigerate for 4 to 6 hours to allow the flavors to marry before serving.
½ cup chopped fresh parsley	
15 ounces canned cannellini beans, rinsed and drained	
¼ cup chopped watercress	
1 tablespoon dried rosemary	
1 tablespoon dried thyme	

Per serving: Calories 186 (From Fat 127); Fat 14g (Saturated 2g); Cholesterol 0mg; Sodium 89mg; Carbohydrate 12g (Dietary Fiber 4g); Protein 3g

Red and Black Bean Salad

Prep time: 10 min • **Cook time:** None • **Yield:** 2 servings

Ingredients	*Directions*
2 tablespoons extra-virgin olive oil	*1* Whisk together the olive oil, honey, balsamic vinegar, lemon juice, and garlic.
1½ tablespoons raw, unprocessed honey	
2 tablespoons balsamic vinegar	*2* Toss the kidney beans and the black beans in the dressing to coat them. Place on two plates and top with pine nuts and basil.
Juice of 1 lemon	
2 cloves garlic, crushed	
15 ounces canned red kidney beans, rinsed and drained	
15 ounces canned black beans, rinsed and drained	
¼ cup pine nuts	
¼ cup chopped fresh basil	

Per serving: Calories 528 (From Fat 210); Fat 23g (Saturated 3g); Cholesterol 0mg; Sodium 498mg; Carbohydrate 62g (Dietary Fiber 16g); Protein 21g

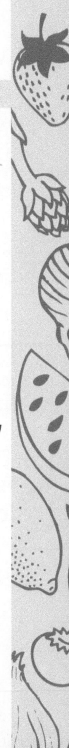

Chapter 13

Making the Main Course: Basic Entrees

*W*ith so many changes in your cupboards and on your menu, is making a main dish that's anti-inflammatory really possible? Definitely! Using seafood, vegetables, and legumes and experimenting with a variety of spices, there's no shortage of main dishes that you can easily make at home.

Once you've set up a menu consisting of the healthiest foods available, make sure you're cooking them correctly. Some methods of cooking — especially grilling, broiling, and, not surprisingly, frying — can actually deplete the vitamins and nutrients in even the healthiest of foods. The best options for healthy cooking are steaming, baking, and poaching; these light cooking methods allow the nutrients to stay put.

In this chapter we look at everyday main dishes, those you can make for your family in relatively little time and with ingredients you're likely to have on hand. All the following recipes combine the healthiest proteins, nutrients, and spices to provide a full meal that helps to prevent or alleviate inflammation.

Packing Vegetarian Dishes Full of Flavor

You may not have given much thought to the various beans in the legume family, but now is a great time to give them a second look. Beans, chickpeas, and other legumes are packed full of fiber, protein, and many other nutrients, all working to help you fight heart disease and some cancers, as well as giving you a sense of being full that helps in weight control.

Combining legumes with seeds, nuts, or grains creates a complete protein, or one that contains all the nine essential amino acids that your body can't make on its own and must get from food sources. That's old news for vegetarians, who don't get any of the essential amino acids from animal sources. But it's also good for meat-eaters to know that they don't have to eat meat at every meal to get the necessary protein levels.

Also included in this group of recipes is tempeh, a fermented soy product and one of the best ways to consume soy other than in the form of edamame. Because it's fermented, tempeh is easy to digest, contains good bacteria, and is high in nutrients and in the cancer- and bone-protective iproflavone components.

Incorporate fermented foods such as fermented beans and dairy products into your diet to get more nutrients and gastrointestinal balancing power out of meals.

Black Bean Burritos

Prep time: 15 min • **Cook time:** None • **Yield:** 4 servings

Ingredients	Directions
Four 10-inch wheat-free or corn-free tortillas	*1* Lay the tortillas flat on separate plates.
1 cup chopped arugula	*2* Sprinkle arugula in a line down the center of each tortilla, leaving about an inch before the edge at both top and bottom.
15 ounces canned black beans, drained	
¼ cup shredded green cabbage	*3* Place equal amounts of black beans, cabbage, avocado, cilantro, and shredded cheese (if desired) on each of the tortillas, following the same line laid out with the arugula. Drizzle a bit of lime juice over the filling.
1 tablespoon lime juice	
1 avocado, peeled, pitted, and sliced	
½ cup chopped fresh cilantro	
6 tablespoons shredded lowfat mozzarella cheese (optional)	*4* Fold the bottom and top inch or so of each tortilla up over the edge of the ingredients; then fold one side of the tortilla over. Roll the burrito so that it's closed.

Per serving: Calories 313 (From Fat 107); Fat 12g (Saturated 2g); Cholesterol 0mg; Sodium 541mg; Carbohydrate 44g (Dietary Fiber 11g); Protein 7g

Tip: Set aside any extra avocado, cabbage, and cheese to use as a topping on the burrito.

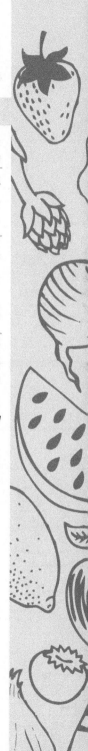

Fava Beans and Artichokes

Prep time: 5 min • **Cook time:** 15 min • **Yield:** 4 servings

Ingredients	*Directions*
1 tablespoon extra-virgin olive oil	*1* Heat the olive oil in a small skillet over medium heat. Sauté the crushed garlic in olive oil for 3 minutes.
2 cloves garlic, crushed	
2 cups shelled fresh or frozen fava beans	*2* Add the fava beans and enough water to barely cover the beans. Cook the beans on medium heat, uncovered, for 7 to 10 minutes or until the beans are cooked and the water is reduced. Remove the beans from the pot.
½ cup artichoke hearts marinated in olive oil	
1 teaspoon dried sage leaves	*3* Mix the beans with the artichoke hearts and marinade, dried sage, and fresh parsley. Season the beans with salt and black pepper.
2 tablespoons chopped fresh flat-leaf parsley	
Sea salt to taste	*4* Serve the beans alone or on top of whole-grain rice (if desired).
Freshly ground black pepper to taste	
2 cups cooked brown rice (optional)	

Per serving: Calories 117 (From Fat 74); Fat 8g (Saturated 1g); Cholesterol 0mg; Sodium 270mg; Carbohydrate 9g (Dietary Fiber 3g); Protein 3g

Beans and Rice with Fennel

Prep time: 10 min plus overnight soak • **Cook time:** 1 hr, 20 min • **Yield:** 6 servings

Ingredients	Directions
8 ounces dried black or white beans (or other beans of your choice)	*1* Soak the beans and seaweed together in water overnight. Discard the water and seaweed and rinse the beans.
1 piece Kombu seaweed	
4 cups water	*2* Bring 4 cups of water to a boil and add the beans and rice, cooking over medium-high heat for about 1 hour. Lower the heat and simmer for 20 minutes. Add more water as needed to prevent the beans and rice from sticking in the pot.
1 cup brown or wild rice	
4 tablespoons extra-virgin olive oil	
1 stalk celery, chopped	*3* When the beans and rice are cooked, remove the seaweed and strain them if needed. Set the beans and rice aside.
1 sweet onion, chopped	
1 cup sliced fresh fennel	
1 cup fresh dill, chopped	*4* In a small bowl, combine the olive oil, celery, onion, fennel, and dill; pour this mix over the beans and rice. Mix well and serve warm.

Per serving: Calories 331 (From Fat 95); Fat 11g (Saturated 2g); Cholesterol 0mg; Sodium 29mg; Carbohydrate 49g (Dietary Fiber 11g); Protein 11g

Tip: Kombu seaweed prevents gas when cooked with beans. It's available in Japanese markets or at various online sales outlets through www.amazon.com.

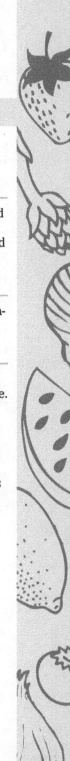

Baked Tempeh and Kale

Prep time: 5 min • **Cook time:** 20–25 min • **Yield:** 2 servings

Ingredients	Directions
8 ounces tempeh, cut into 1-inch pieces	**1** Preheat the oven to 350 degrees.
½ cup chopped onion	**2** In a medium saucepan, bring the vegetable broth to a boil over medium-high heat. Add the tempeh and onion and boil for 5 minutes.
½ cup organic vegetable broth	
½ cup sliced mushrooms	
1 teaspoon turmeric	**3** Transfer the boiled tempeh and onions along with the remaining broth to a glass baking dish. Add the sliced mushrooms, turmeric, cumin, and sesame seeds to the tempeh and stir well. Bake for 15 minutes.
1 teaspoon cumin	
2 tablespoons sesame seeds	
1 cup kale, chopped	**4** Add the kale to the dish and bake for another 5 minutes.
1 tablespoon wheat-free tamari sauce	
2 tablespoons nutritional yeast	**5** Remove the tempeh from the oven. Season the tempeh with tamari sauce and sprinkle it with nutritional yeast.

Per serving: Calories 308 (From Fat 129); Fat 14g (Saturated 2g); Cholesterol 0mg; Sodium 669mg; Carbohydrate 23g (Dietary Fiber 9g); Protein 25g

Note: *Nutritional yeast* is a deactivated yeast used by many vegans and vegetarians as a seasoning or food enhancement. With its nutty, cheesy flavor, it's often sprinkled on hot popcorn or garlic bread.

Escarole and White Beans

Prep time: 5 min • **Cook time:** 20 min • **Yield:** 5 servings

Ingredients	*Directions*
3 tablespoons extra-virgin olive oil	*1* Heat the olive oil in a large sauté pan over medium heat. Add the garlic, red pepper flakes, and marjoram. Add the escarole in batches, letting each batch cook down a bit to make room for more in the pan. Cook for approximately 10 minutes, stirring occasionally.
2 cloves garlic, crushed	
½ teaspoon crushed red pepper flakes	
1 teaspoon crushed dried marjoram	*2* Add the broth and wine along with the white beans. Cook the beans for another 10 minutes or until they're warm. Sprinkle the beans with parsley and season with salt and black pepper. Serve the beans over brown rice or risotto.
2 heads escarole	
¼ cup organic vegetable broth or chicken broth	
2 tablespoons dry white wine	
15 ounces canned cannellini beans, rinsed and drained	
2 tablespoons chopped fresh parsley	
Sea salt to taste	
Freshly ground black pepper to taste	
1 cup cooked brown rice or Arborio rice	

Per serving: Calories 200 (From Fat 83); Fat 9g (Saturated 1g); Cholesterol 0mg; Sodium 257mg; Carbohydrate 25g (Dietary Fiber 10g); Protein 6g

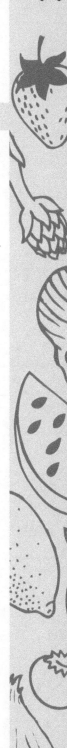

Quinoa and Black Beans with Swiss Chard

Prep time: 10 min • **Cook time:** 10–15 min • **Yield:** 4 servings

Ingredients	Directions
1 cup uncooked quinoa	*1* Rinse and strain the quinoa in water; set the quinoa aside.
1 teaspoon extra-virgin olive oil	
2 cloves garlic, minced	*2* Heat the olive oil in a large sauté pan over medium heat. Sauté the minced garlic in the olive oil for about 30 seconds until lightly browned. Add the Swiss chard and stir for 1 to 2 minutes.
2 cups Swiss chard	
15 ounces canned black beans, rinsed and drained	
1 cup vegetable broth	*3* Add the strained quinoa, black beans, vegetable broth, coconut milk, and curry powder to the garlic. Reduce the heat and simmer for 10 to 15 minutes.
½ cup coconut milk	
1 teaspoon curry powder	
½ cup chopped fresh cilantro	*4* Top the quinoa with chopped cilantro and scallions.
2 scallions, chopped	

Per serving: Calories 307 (From Fat 96); Fat 11g (Saturated 6g); Cholesterol 0mg; Sodium 289mg; Carbohydrate 44g (Dietary Fiber 8g); Protein 11g

Serving Up Chicken and Seafood Entrees

Chicken is often thought of as a healthy alternative to red meat, but that's only true if you choose your chicken well. A piece of dark meat, such as a drumstick, with the skin on can be fairly high in fat. A 4-ounce serving of skinless white meat has two-thirds of the daily recommendation of protein and is your best choice when looking for anti-inflammatory benefits.

Seafood has all the benefits of chicken and more; many fish, like salmon and mackerel, contain high levels of omega-3 fatty acid, an essential fatty acid that helps raise the HDL — or *good* — cholesterol levels in your body. Keeping the HDL at a manageable level can help prevent cardiovascular disease.

While chicken and seafood are high in protein, they don't contain the fiber and phytonutrients found in beans, so we recommend that you balance chicken and seafood entrees with bean and legume dishes (refer to the recipes in the previous section).

The recipes in this section use the best of chicken and seafood in a variety of ways meant to feed the average family and help fight inflammation.

Roasted Lemon Chicken with Broccoli

Prep time: 20 min • **Cook time:** 40–45 min • **Yield:** 8 servings

Ingredients	Directions
1 whole raw organic chicken (3–4 pounds)	**1** Preheat the oven to 400 degrees. Lightly oil a small roasting pan.
2 tablespoons extra-virgin olive oil	**2** In a small bowl, combine 1 tablespoon of the olive oil with the thyme, oregano, juice from one lemon, salt, and black pepper. Save the used lemon rind.
1 tablespoon dried thyme	
1 tablespoon dried oregano	
2 lemons	**3** Remove the giblets from the chicken's body cavity (discard them or use them for another recipe). Rinse the chicken under cold water and pat it dry with a towel. Rub the chicken with the olive-oil mixture and place the used lemon rind in the cavity of the chicken.
1 teaspoon sea salt	
1 teaspoon freshly ground black pepper	
1 onion, chopped	**4** Place the chopped onion in the bottom of the roasting pan, and set the chicken on top. Cook the chicken for 40 to 50 minutes or until the internal temperature reads at least 165 degrees with meat thermometer inserted in the chicken's inner thigh.
½ cup water	
4 cups broccoli spears	
4 sprigs parsley, chopped	
	5 When the chicken has about 10 minutes left to bake, bring the water to a boil in saucepan with a steamer basket set inside. Set the broccoli in the steamer and steam until it is fork tender but still green.
	6 Top the broccoli with remaining 1 tablespoon olive oil, chopped parsley, and the juice of the other lemon. Serve the broccoli alongside the roasted chicken and onions.

Per serving: Calories 250 (From Fat 139); Fat 15g (Saturated 4g); Cholesterol 67mg; Sodium 363mg; Carbohydrate 5g (Dietary Fiber 2g); Protein 23g

Creamy Chicken Curry

Prep time: 5–7 min • **Cook time:** 10–20 min • **Yield:** 8 servings

Ingredients	Directions
2 tablespoons extra-virgin olive oil	**1** Heat the olive oil in a large skillet over medium heat. Sauté the onions and the bay leaf in the olive oil until the onions are slightly translucent, about 5 minutes. Add the garlic in the last minute of cooking.
2 onions, chopped	
1 bay leaf	
2 cloves garlic, minced	**2** Add the chicken to the skillet and cook until it's no longer pink on the outside.
1 pound raw boneless, skinless chicken breast, cut into 1-inch cubes	
15 ounces coconut milk	**3** Add the coconut milk, peas, chopped broccoli, curry powder, chili powder, and paprika to the skillet. Cook until the chicken is done, about 7 minutes. Remove the bay leaf.
1 cup fresh or frozen peas	
1 cup chopped broccoli	
2 teaspoons curry powder	
2 teaspoons chili powder	**4** Top the chicken with cilantro and serve with steamed brown rice, quinoa, or millet.
1 tablespoon paprika	
½ cup fresh chopped cilantro	
4 cups cooked brown rice, quinoa, or millet	

Per serving: Calories 343 (From Fat 154); Fat 17g (Saturated 11g); Cholesterol 31mg; Sodium 54mg; Carbohydrate 33g (Dietary Fiber 6g); Protein 17g

Pesto Pasta with Salmon

Prep time: 15 min • **Cook time:** 15 min • **Yield:** 6 servings

Ingredients	*Directions*
16 ounces brown rice pasta	*1* Cook the pasta in boiling water as directed on the package. Drain the pasta and place it in a large bowl.
3 tablespoons pesto (see the following recipe)	
2 cups flaked cooked wild Pacific sockeye salmon	*2* Add the pesto to the cooked pasta and stir to combine.
1 cup baby spinach	*3* Top the pasta with spinach and salmon, and sprinkle with Parmesan cheese (if desired).
1 tablespoon freshly grated Parmesan cheese (optional)	

Pesto

1 cup fresh basil leaves	*1* Combine the basil, garlic, and pine nuts or walnuts in a food processor. Drizzle in the olive oil while the basil mixture processes. You can store the pesto in the refrigerator for up to a week.
3 cloves crushed garlic	
1 tablespoon pine nuts or walnuts	
2 tablespoons extra-virgin olive oil	

Per serving: Calories 378 (From Fat 53); Fat 6g (Saturated 1g); Cholesterol 34mg; Sodium 32mg; Carbohydrate 57g (Dietary Fiber 2g); Protein 17g

Tip: Vital Choice (www.vitalchoice.com) is a good online source for low-toxicity canned salmon.

Marinated Broiled Salmon with Steamed Broccoli

Prep time: 5 min • **Cook time:** 10–15 min • **Yield:** 4 servings

Ingredients	Directions
2 tablespoons extra-virgin olive oil	*1* Position the oven rack so it's a few inches below the broiler at the top of the oven. Preheat the broiler.
Four 8-ounce salmon fillets	
½ inch piece fresh ginger	*2* Drizzle a glass baking dish for the salmon with 1 tablespoon of the olive oil. Place the salmon fillets in the dish. Peel the ginger and grate it over the salmon fillets.
¼ cup dry white wine	
2 lemons	
½ cup water	*3* Add the dry white wine and juice of one lemon to the baking dish.
4 cups broccoli spears	
Sea salt to taste	*4* Broil the salmon for 7 to 10 minutes or until it's translucent.
4 tablespoons fresh flat-leaf parsley	
2 cups brown rice or quinoa	*5* While the salmon is broiling, bring the water to a boil in saucepan with a steamer basket set inside. Set the broccoli in the steamer and steam until it is fork tender but still green. Transfer the broccoli to a serving dish and drizzle with the remaining 1 tablespoon olive oil and the juice of half the remaining lemon; season with salt.
	6 Remove the salmon from the oven. Top the salmon with parsley and the juice of the remaining half lemon. Serve the salmon with the steamed broccoli and brown rice or quinoa.

Per serving: Calories 482 (From Fat 148); Fat 16g (Saturated 3g); Cholesterol 129mg; Sodium 336mg; Carbohydrate 28g (Dietary Fiber 4g); Protein 54g

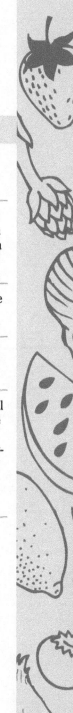

Baked Cod over Spinach

Prep time: 10 min • **Cook time:** 10–25 min • **Yield:** 4 servings

Ingredients	Directions
1 clove garlic, crushed	**1** Preheat the oven to 375 degrees. Lightly oil a glass baking dish.
1 teaspoon dried oregano	
1 tablespoon extra-virgin olive oil	**2** Combine the garlic, oregano, olive-oil, lemon zest, and black pepper in a shallow bowl or plate. Dip the cod fillets in the olive-oil mixture and place them in the glass baking dish.
1 teaspoon lemon zest	
1 teaspoon freshly ground black pepper	
4 cod fillets	**3** Bake the cod fillets for 15 to 20 minutes or until they're flaky.
2 cups baby spinach	
2 tablespoons fresh chopped parsley	**4** Lay a bed of spinach on the plate and top with a cod fillet. Sprinkle the cod with chopped parsley, and serve the lemon wedges on the side.
1 lemon, cut in wedges	

Per serving: Calories 232 (From Fat 45); Fat 5g (Saturated 1g); Cholesterol 99mg; Sodium 162mg; Carbohydrate 4g (Dietary Fiber 1g); Protein 42g

Tip: For a little extra zest, squeeze a bit of lemon juice over the bed of spinach before topping it with the cod.

Bean and Tuna Lettuce Wraps

Prep time: 15 min • **Cook time:** None • **Yield:** 4–6 servings

Ingredients	*Directions*
2 tablespoons Dijon mustard	*1* Whisk together the Dijon mustard, olive oil, yogurt (if desired), and lemon juice.
4 tablespoons extra-virgin olive oil	
1 tablespoon plain Greek yogurt, 0–2% fat (optional)	*2* Add the beans, tuna, onion, parsley, cilantro, celery, and carrot to the mustard mixture, and mix well.
2 tablespoons lemon juice	
3 cups cooked beans (any kind)	*3* Wash, dry, and arrange the lettuce leaves on a plate. Scoop the bean mixture into the lettuce leaves and roll them up, tucking the sides inside.
1 cup canned tuna in water, drained	
1 medium onion, diced	
¼ cup chopped fresh parsley	
¼ cup chopped fresh cilantro	
2 celery stalks, diced	
1 carrot, diced	
1 small head of whole butter lettuce leaves, separated	

Per serving: Calories 375 (From Fat 145); Fat 16g (Saturated 2g); Cholesterol 15mg; Sodium 367mg; Carbohydrate 38g (Dietary Fiber 11g); Protein 22g

Vary It! For a variety of tastes, vary the wrap with Romaine and other lettuce types, or add a few spinach leaves.

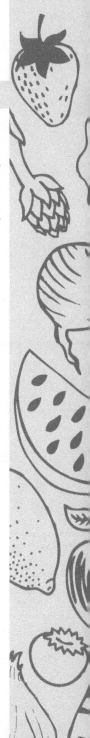

Halibut with Green Beans

Prep time: 10 min • **Cook time:** 20 min • **Yield:** 4 servings

Ingredients	Directions
2 tablespoons extra-virgin olive oil, divided	*1* Preheat the oven to 375 degrees.
8 ounces fresh green beans	*2* In a glass baking dish, drizzle the green beans with a little olive oil and bake for 20 minutes.
1 medium onion, sliced	
Four 6-ounce halibut steaks	*3* Pour 1 tablespoon of the olive oil in the bottom of another glass baking dish, place the onion on top, and then place the halibut steaks on top of the onions. Drizzle the remaining olive oil over the top of the fish. Add the fish to the oven to bake alongside the green beans for the last 15 minutes.
¼ cup fresh dill, chopped	
Juice of 1 lemon	
1 teaspoon kelp, crumbled or flaked	
Sea salt to taste	*4* After removing the fish from the oven, add the chopped dill, lemon juice, kelp, and salt and black pepper to taste. Serve with brown rice and the green beans on the side.
Freshly ground black pepper to taste	
2 cups cooked brown rice	

Per serving: Calories 367 (From Fat 97); Fat 11g (Saturated 1g); Cholesterol 53mg; Sodium 98mg; Carbohydrate 30g (Dietary Fiber 4g); Protein 39g

Note: Kelp and other forms of seaweed have many health benefits, helping to strengthen the immune system as well as serving as a pain reliever for minor irritants.

Chapter 14

Cranking Your Entrees Up a Notch

*N*o matter what your lifestyle, you sometimes just want something nice for dinner — something that goes a bit beyond the everyday foods that seem to end up on your planner every week. But how far can you go when it comes to nice cooking when you're living an anti-inflammatory lifestyle? You may be surprised.

The kinds of foods you eat are only part of the problem in terms of eating right; how that food is prepared is another big thing to consider when you want your diet to mirror your lifestyle. That piece of fish you have in your refrigerator is going to work much better for you if you pan sear it or broil it than if you fry it — and it's going to retain most of its natural flavors and vitamins and nutrients.

The recipes in this chapter go beyond the ordinary, everyday menu and offer many options for entertaining at home. Many are made with less common ingredients that may require a trip to the store. These entrees are specially designed for entertaining at home, whether you're cooking for friends, hosting dinner with the boss, or just marking the celebration of a special occasion.

Making Main Dishes Special

Usually, transforming any dish from mundane to magnificent just takes a little creativity. Take a lean cut of meat, a piece of poultry, or a hearty seafood steak and give it a walnut crust, infuse it with herbs and spices, or simply dress it up with a flavorful marinade. These flourishes can not only turn a meal from drab to daring but also add a stronger anti-inflammatory boost because many herbs, nuts, and seeds carry inflammation-fighting properties of their own.

In general, choose grass-fed, organic, and free-range varieties of meats and seafood that are low in mercury. These meats are healthier because they're leaner (they have less saturated fat), have more of the good fats, are more nutrient dense, and don't contain the toxins found in non-organic, mass-produced varieties. Your local butcher, health food or whole food store, and www.localharvest.org are some resources for finding the best and least inflammatory sources of meat, poultry, and seafood.

Adding herbs and spices to your food increases its antioxidant value. The essential oils in dried herbs are more highly concentrated than in fresh, so you should use less dried herbs for flavoring than you would use fresh. The conversion is as simple as switching from tablespoons to teaspoons: For example, if a recipe calls for 2 tablespoons fresh herbs, use 2 teaspoons dried.

Walnut-Encrusted Salmon Steaks

Prep time: 45 min • **Cook time:** 15–20 min • **Yield:** 4 servings

Ingredients	*Directions*
1 cup walnuts	*1* Combine the walnuts, orange zest, ginger, and 2 tablespoons of the olive oil in a food processor and pulse to a coarse consistency.
1 tablespoon orange zest	
1 teaspoon ground ginger	
4 tablespoons extra-virgin olive oil, divided	*2* Brush the salmon fillets with the Dijon mustard, and then coat the fillets with the walnut mixture. Refrigerate the salmon fillets for at least 30 minutes before baking.
4 salmon fillets	
2 tablespoons Dijon mustard	
2 cups Brussels sprouts, washed and halved	*3* Preheat the oven to 350 degrees. Place the Brussels sprouts around the sides of a roasting pan, leaving room for the salmon fillets. Drizzle the sprouts with the remaining 2 tablespoons olive oil.
1 lemon, cut into wedges	
	4 Bake the Brussels sprouts on their own for 12 minutes before taking the pan out of the oven and adding the salmon fillets to the center of the pan.
	5 Bake the salmon and Brussels sprouts together for 12 to 15 minutes until the salmon is flaky. Serve with lemon wedges.

Per serving: Calories 685 (From Fat 375); Fat 42g (Saturated 5g); Cholesterol 166mg; Sodium 414mg; Carbohydrate 10g (Dietary Fiber 3g); Protein 69g

Note: Brussels sprouts are full of phytonutrients — natural plant compounds — which are believed to help prevent cancer. They're also full of fiber, vitamins A and C, potassium, folate, and iron and help the liver to detoxify your body of harmful substances.

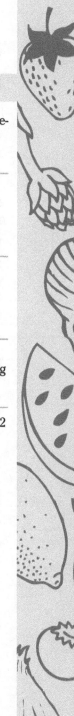

Tilapia with Daikon Radish and Bean Sprouts over Brown Rice

Prep time: 15 min • **Cook time:** 45 min • **Yield:** 4 servings

Ingredients	Directions
2 cups water	**1** Boil the water and add the brown rice. Reduce the heat and simmer, covered, for 40 minutes or until the rice is cooked.
1 cup brown rice	
5 tablespoons sesame oil	
3 tablespoons rice wine vinegar	**2** Preheat the oven to 350 degrees. Whisk together the sesame oil, rice wine vinegar, umeboshi plum paste, tamari sauce, agave nectar, and chopped cilantro to make a dressing. Toss the daikon radish and the bean sprouts in the dressing.
2 tablespoons umeboshi plum paste	
1½ teaspoons wheat-free tamari sauce	
¾ teaspoon agave nectar	**3** Place the tilapia in a baking dish. Combine the ginger and cayenne pepper in a small bowl. Drizzle the olive oil over the tilapia and sprinkle with the ginger mixture. Bake for 10 to 15 minutes or until the inside of the fish is no longer translucent.
3 tablespoons chopped fresh cilantro	
1 daikon radish, peeled and finely sliced	
2 cups bean sprouts	**4** Serve over brown rice, topped with the daikon radish and bean sprouts. Garnish with lime wedges.
1 pound tilapia fillets	
1 teaspoon peeled, minced ginger	
½ teaspoon cayenne pepper	
1 teaspoon extra-virgin olive oil	
1 lime, cut into wedges	

Per serving: Calories 472 (From Fat 199); Fat 22g (Saturated 4g); Cholesterol 49mg; Sodium 751mg; Carbohydrate 43g (Dietary Fiber 5g); Protein 28g

Tip: You can find umeboshi plum paste in some natural food stores or Asian food stores. It's also available online at places such as www.amazon.com or www.vitacost.com.

Tuna Steaks with Citrus Dressing over Quinoa

Prep time: 30 min • **Cook time:** 45 min • **Yield:** 4 servings

Ingredients	Directions
2 cups quinoa	*1* Rinse the quinoa in cold water and drain it. Bring the quinoa to a boil in 3½ cups water, and then reduce the heat and simmer for 20 minutes.
3½ cups water	
Four 6-ounce tuna steaks	
1 shallot, chopped	*2* In a large skillet, bring 1½ to 2 inches of water to a boil and set a steamer basket on top. Place the tuna steaks and shallots in the steamer basket and cover; steam for about 6 to 8 minutes.
2 grapefruits	
¼ cup white wine vinegar	
1 tablespoon fresh ginger, chopped	*3* Whisk together the juice of one grapefruit, white wine vinegar, ginger, and olive oil. Set the mix aside.
2 tablespoons extra-virgin olive oil	
2 cups fresh green beans, ends removed and beans snapped in half	*4* Steam the green beans covered in a pan with a little water for 5 minutes or until they're softened but still bright green. Toss the green beans with the grapefruit dressing.
1 seedless tangerine, peeled and separated into segments	*5* Dish up the cooked quinoa first. Then add the green beans and top with the tuna steaks. Garnish with tangerine slices, the fruit of the second grapefruit, and sliced almonds.
2 tablespoons sliced almonds	

Per serving: Calories 647 (From Fat 136); Fat 15g (Saturated 2g); Cholesterol 74mg; Sodium 82mg; Carbohydrate 77g (Dietary Fiber 9g); Protein 52g

Vary It! If you're sensitive to citrus, you can substitute ½ cup chopped pineapple for the grapefruit juice and omit the grapefruit and tangerine garnishes.

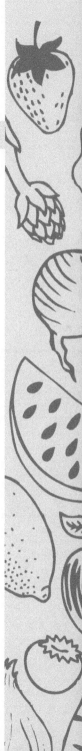

Baked Halibut with Cajun Spices and Collard Greens

Prep time: 30 min • **Cook time:** 45 min • **Yield:** 2 servings

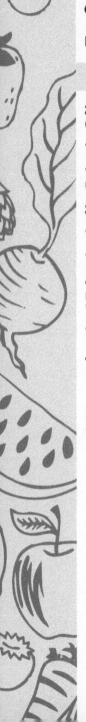

Ingredients	Directions
2 tablespoons extra-virgin olive oil, divided	*1* Preheat the oven to 400 degrees. Combine 1 tablespoon of the olive oil, dill, and 1 tablespoon of the Old Bay Seasoning; rub on both sides of the halibut.
1 tablespoon dried dill	
1 tablespoon plus ½ teaspoon Old Bay Seasoning, divided	*2* Place the tomato (if desired) and onion in a lightly oiled baking pan. Put the seasoned fillets in the baking pan and bake for 10 minutes or until the fish is cooked.
2 halibut fillets	
1 tomato, diced (optional)	
1 small onion, chopped	*3* While the fish bakes, put the collard greens in a saucepan with ½ cup water and bring to a boil. Reduce the heat and simmer, covered, for about 5 minutes.
4 ounces collard greens, rib removed and chopped into 1-inch pieces	
½ cup water	*4* Put the collard greens in a medium bowl with the remaining 1 tablespoon olive oil, lemon juice, and the remaining ½ teaspoon of Old Bay Seasoning. Mix well and serve the greens alongside the halibut, onion, and tomato.
Juice of 1 lemon	

Per serving: Calories 599 (From Fat 209); Fat 23g (Saturated 3g); Cholesterol 130mg; Sodium 629mg; Carbohydrate 8g (Dietary Fiber 3g); Protein 87g

Salmon and Avocado Sushi Roll

Prep time: 45 min • **Cook time:** 35–45 min • **Yield:** 6 servings

Ingredients	*Directions*
1 cup short-grain sushi rice	**1** Thoroughly rinse the sushi rice. Add the rice to a cup of water in a saucepan. Bring the water to a boil, and then reduce heat and simmer the rice, covered, until cooked, 35 to 40 minutes.
1 cup water	
1 tablespoon rice wine vinegar	
8 Nori seaweed sheets	**2** Add the rice wine vinegar to the cooked rice and mix together gently. Set the rice aside to cool before assembling the sushi rolls.
2 tablespoons sesame seeds	
6 ounces gravlax or smoked salmon, very thinly sliced	**3** Place the Nori sheets on a flat surface, sprinkle each sheet with water, and add 3 tablespoons of sushi rice to the middle of each sheet, spreading it thinly and gently pressing it into the Nori.
1 avocado, peeled, pitted, and thinly sliced	
½ cup bean sprouts	
1-inch piece daikon radish, cut into matchstick strips	**4** Sprinkle sesame seeds on top of the rice and along one edge of the Nori sheet. Evenly divide the salmon, avocado, bean sprouts, daikon radish, and cucumber on top of each Nori and rice sheet.
½ cucumber, peeled and thinly sliced	
1 tablespoon wheat-free tamari sauce	**5** Use a sushi roller or bamboo mat to roll the Nori sheet into a log, keeping the ingredients rolled as tightly as possible. Sprinkle water on the layers as you roll if they're not sticking together.
Wasabi paste to taste	
Pickled ginger slices	
	6 Slice the roll into 1-inch rounds using a sharp knife dipped in water. Place the sushi roll rounds on a plate.
	7 Mix the tamari sauce with a little wasabi to taste (or dab a little wasabi directly on a sushi round) and use the tamari sauce for lightly dipping the sushi rounds. Serve the sushi with ginger slices.

Per serving: Calories 195 (From Fat 62); Fat 7g (Saturated 1g); Cholesterol 7mg; Sodium 841mg; Carbohydrate 25g (Dietary Fiber 4g); Protein 9g

Sardines and Olives over Spiced Wild Rice

Prep time: 20 min • **Cook time:** 30–45 min • **Yield:** 4 servings

Ingredients	Directions
1 cup whole-grain wild rice mixture	*1* Rinse and drain the wild rice. Bring the broth and water to a boil in a saucepan, and add the rice. Reduce the heat and simmer, covered, until the rice is cooked, 30 to 45 minutes.
1 cup organic chicken broth	
2 cups water	
2 scallions, chopped	*2* Let the rice cool for a few minutes and then transfer it to a bowl. Add the scallions, olives, cilantro, and the pine nuts and mix together.
¼ cup Kalamata olives	
½ cup chopped fresh cilantro	
3 tablespoons pine nuts	*3* In a small bowl, whisk together the lemon juice, olive oil, cayenne pepper, and curry powder. Pour this dressing over the rice mixture and stir gently.
Juice of 1 lemon	
3 tablespoons extra-virgin olive oil	
½ teaspoon ground cayenne red pepper	*4* Evenly divide the baby spinach on each plate and spoon the rice mixture onto the spinach. Top the rice mixture with the sardines and sprinkle with feta cheese (if desired).
1 tablespoon curry powder	
4 cups baby spinach	
Two 4-ounce cans sardines	
¼ cup feta cheese (optional)	

Per serving: Calories 459 (From Fat 239); Fat 27g (Saturated 5g); Cholesterol 68mg; Sodium 1,062mg; Carbohydrate 40g (Dietary Fiber 3g); Protein 19g

Ginger Salmon Burgers with Arugula

Prep time: 15 min • **Cook time:** 10–20 min • **Yield:** 4 servings

Ingredients	Directions
2 tablespoons extra-virgin olive oil	*1* Preheat the oven to 350 degrees. Whisk together the olive oil, ginger, mustard, and 2 tablespoons of the lemon juice. Drizzle this mixture over the salmon burgers.
1 teaspoon ground ginger	
1 teaspoon dry mustard	
Juice of 1 lemon, divided	*2* Bake the salmon burgers for 8 to 10 minutes, flipping them halfway through the cooking time.
4 salmon burgers	
1 tomato, chopped	*3* Toss the tomato, arugula, parsley, and artichoke hearts in the remaining lemon juice, and top the burgers with the mixture.
2 cups arugula, chopped	
¼ cup chopped fresh parsley	
1 cup marinated artichoke hearts	

Per serving: Calories 280 (From Fat 162); Fat 18g (Saturated 2g); Cholesterol 60mg; Sodium 462mg; Carbohydrate 9g (Dietary Fiber 2g); Protein 22g

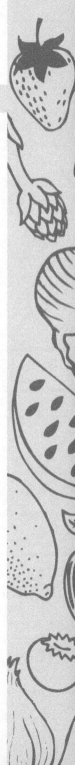

Curried Chicken with Broccoli

Prep time: 20 min • **Cook time:** 30 min • **Yield:** 4 servings

Ingredients	Directions
3 tablespoons extra-virgin olive oil	*1* Heat the olive oil in a large skillet over medium heat; add the garlic, onion, bay leaf, curry powder, paprika, cayenne pepper, ginger, and chicken and cook for 10 to 15 minutes, until the chicken is lightly browned.
3 cloves garlic, chopped	
1 onion, chopped	
1 bay leaf	
3 tablespoons curry powder	*2* Add the broccoli and coconut milk, and simmer for 5 minutes.
1 tablespoon paprika	
½ teaspoon ground red cayenne pepper	*3* Reduce the heat and stir in the yogurt. Cook over low heat for another 5 minutes. Serve over brown rice.
1 teaspoon fresh grated ginger	
2 boneless, skinless chicken breasts cut into bite-sized pieces	
2 cups broccoli florets	
¾ cup coconut milk	
1 cup plain yogurt, 0–2% fat	
4 cups cooked brown rice	

Per serving: Calories 555 (From Fat 223); Fat 25g (Saturated 11g); Cholesterol 40mg; Sodium 104mg; Carbohydrate 61g (Dietary Fiber 8g); Protein 25g

Tip: If you're sensitive to foods in the nightshade family — tomatoes, eggplant, potatoes, sweet peppers, and hot peppers — you should omit the paprika from this recipe. Nightshade vegetable sensitivity can affect nerve and joint health.

Spiced Chicken with Turnips and Cabbage

Prep time: 15 min • **Cook time:** 40–50 min • **Yield:** 6 servings

Ingredients	*Directions*
1 tablespoon ground mustard	*1* Preheat the oven to 400 degrees. Combine the ground mustard, turmeric, dill, and olive oil. Place the chicken in a baking dish and rub the chicken with this mixture.
1 teaspoon turmeric	
1 teaspoon ground dill seed	
2 tablespoons extra-virgin olive oil	
1 whole organic chicken, rinsed and dried, with giblets removed	*2* Arrange the turnips, cabbage, shallots, and leek around the chicken in the baking dish. Cook the chicken for 40 to 50 minutes or until the internal temperature reads at least 165 degrees with meat thermometer inserted in the chicken's inner thigh.
2 turnips, chopped	
2 cups cabbage, chopped	*3* Dress the chicken with lemon juice and chopped dill. Serve it with quinoa, millet, or whole-grain rice.
2 shallots, sliced	
1 leek, rinsed well and chopped	
Juice of 1 lemon	
¼ cup fresh chopped dill weed	
3 cups cooked quinoa, millet, or whole-grain rice	

Per serving: Calories 540 (From Fat 245); Fat 27g (Saturated 7g); Cholesterol 122mg; Sodium 219mg; Carbohydrate 30g (Dietary Fiber 3g); Protein 43g

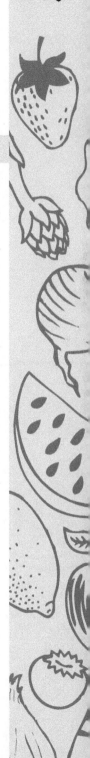

Coconut Chicken with Beet and Cabbage Slaw

Prep time: 30 min • **Cook time:** 30 min • **Yield:** 6 servings

Ingredients	Directions
2 raw beets, peeled	*1* In a saucepan with about ½ cup water, steam the beets about 15 minutes, making sure they remain firm but are able to be pierced with a fork. Let them cool for a few minutes and then shred them with a food processor or hand shredder.
1½ pounds boneless, skinless chicken breast, cubed	
1 tablespoon curry powder	
6 tablespoons extra-virgin olive oil, divided	*2* As the beets steam, prepare the chicken by tossing it with the curry powder.
1 onion, chopped	
2 cups shredded cabbage	*3* Heat 2 tablespoons of olive oil in a large skillet over medium heat. Add the onion and cook until it's translucent, about 5 minutes.
2 tablespoons apple cider vinegar	
1 teaspoon caraway seed	*4* Add the chicken pieces and cook for 5 more minutes.
One 14-ounce can coconut milk	*5* Add the coconut milk to the skillet and let the chicken simmer until cooked, about 15 to 20 minutes.
2 tablespoons shredded organic coconut	
	6 Combine the remaining 4 tablespoons of olive oil, shredded beets, cabbage, cider vinegar, caraway seed, and shredded coconut. Serve the cabbage slaw alongside the chicken.

Per serving: Calories 429 (From Fat 287); Fat 32g (Saturated 16g); Cholesterol 63mg; Sodium 112mg; Carbohydrate 12g (Dietary Fiber 4g); Protein 26g

Note: Coconut has long been regarded as a valuable health aid. People in ancient times used coconut to treat toothaches, abscesses, baldness, and bronchitis, among other ailments. Modern medicine hails its use against bacteria that cause ulcers and urinary tract infections; it's also a source of quick energy and a digestive aid.

Chicken with Greek Yogurt Sauce

Prep time: 10 min • **Cook time:** 20–30 min • **Yield:** 6 servings

Ingredients	Directions
2 tablespoons extra-virgin olive oil	**1** Heat the olive oil in a large skillet over medium heat. Cook the chicken and onion in the olive oil until the chicken is lightly browned and cooked through, about 15 minutes. Remove the skillet from the heat and let the chicken cool.
1 pound boneless, skinless chicken breasts, cubed	
1 onion, chopped	
2 cloves garlic, minced	**2** In a large bowl, combine the garlic, cucumber, parsley, mint, yogurt, and lemon juice. Toss the cooled chicken in the sauce.
1 cucumber, chopped	
¼ cup chopped fresh parsley	
1 teaspoon chopped fresh mint	**3** Serve the chicken with brown rice or quinoa and a side of steamed broccoli.
½ cup plain Greek yogurt, 0–2% fat	
1 tablespoon fresh lemon juice	
3 cups cooked brown rice or quinoa	
3 cups steamed broccoli	

Per serving: Calories 281 (From Fat 71); Fat 8g (Saturated 2g); Cholesterol 43mg; Sodium 71mg; Carbohydrate 31g (Dietary Fiber 5g); Protein 22g

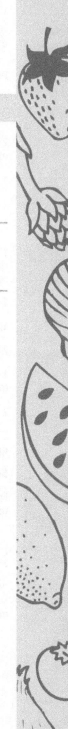

Baked Chicken with Mushrooms

Prep time: 10 min • **Cook time:** 40–50 min • **Yield:** 4 servings

Ingredients	*Directions*
2 tablespoons plus 1 teaspoon extra-virgin olive oil, divided 1 tablespoon dried sage 1 tablespoon dried oregano 2 cloves garlic, minced 1 whole organic chicken, rinsed and dried, with giblets removed 1 onion, chopped 1 head bok choy, chopped 2 stalks of celery, chopped 1 red bell pepper, chopped (optional) 2 cups mushrooms, sliced 2 cups cooked brown rice or quinoa Sea salt to taste Freshly ground black pepper to taste	*1* Preheat the oven to 400 degrees. Combine 2 tablespoons olive oil, sage, oregano, and garlic and rub the mixture over the chicken. *2* Lightly oil a small roasting pan. Put the onions, bok choy, celery, red bell pepper (if desired), and mushrooms in a bowl and toss with 1 teaspoon olive oil; then transfer to the roasting pan and place the chicken on top. *3* Cook the chicken for 40 to 50 minutes or until the internal temperature reads at least 165 degrees with meat thermometer inserted in the chicken's inner thigh. *4* Serve the chicken with brown rice or quinoa. Salt and pepper the chicken and vegetables to taste.

Per serving: Calories 777 (From Fat 375); Fat 42g (Saturated 10g); Cholesterol 182mg; Sodium 487mg; Carbohydrate 35g (Dietary Fiber 6g); Protein 65g

Note: Bok choy, or Chinese cabbage, is a cruciferous vegetable like broccoli, cauliflower, and Brussels sprouts. It may help prevent some cancers, particularly lung, colon, prostate, and endometrial (uterine) cancers.

Sweet Baked Lamb with Butternut Squash

Prep time: 10 min • **Cook time:** 1 hr • **Yield:** 6 servings

Ingredients	Directions
1 tablespoon extra-virgin olive oil	*1* Preheat the oven to 400 degrees and lightly oil a 9-x-13 baking dish.
½ teaspoon cinnamon	
1 tablespoon dried thyme	*2* Combine the olive oil with the cinnamon, thyme, crushed garlic, and black pepper. Rub this mixture on the lamb shanks.
1 clove garlic, crushed	
1 teaspoon freshly ground black pepper	
6 lamb shanks or leg of lamb	*3* Place the shallots, onion, carrots, and butternut squash in the bottom of the baking dish. Place the seasoned lamb shanks on top of the vegetable mixture. Add the water. Cover the pan and bake the lamb for approximately 40 minutes; then bake uncovered for an additional 20 minutes.
2 shallots, diced	
1 sweet onion, chopped	
1 cup carrots, chopped	
1 butternut squash, peeled, deseeded, and cut into 1-inch pieces	
½ cup water	

Per serving: Calories 396 (From Fat 129); Fat 14g (Saturated 5g); Cholesterol 156mg; Sodium 135mg; Carbohydrate 13g (Dietary Fiber 3g); Protein 52g

Note: Lamb tends to be a hypoallergenic meat, but it's still a red meat, so it may not be suitable for everyone following an anti-inflammation diet.

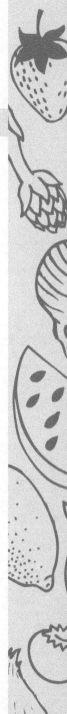

Turkey Meatballs over Rice

Prep time: 15 min • **Cook time:** 40 min • **Yield:** 6 servings

Ingredients	Directions
1½ cups whole-grain rice mix	*1* Rinse and drain the rice. Bring the water to a boil in a small saucepan and add the rice. Reduce the heat, and simmer, covered, for 20 to 30 minutes or until the rice is cooked.
2½ cups water	
1 pound ground turkey	
1 egg	*2* While the rice cooks, combine the ground turkey, egg, crushed crackers, thyme, salt, and black pepper in a large bowl.
¼ cup crushed savory rice crackers	
1 teaspoon dried thyme	
1 teaspoon sea salt	*3* Heat the olive oil in a large saucepan over medium heat. Sauté the garlic and onion until the onion is almost transparent, about 5 minutes.
1 tablespoon freshly ground black pepper	
3 tablespoons extra-virgin olive oil	*4* Form the turkey mixture into 1-inch balls and place the meatballs in the pan with the onions and garlic. Cook the meatballs for 20 minutes, turning them periodically to ensure that they're browned on all sides.
½ onion, chopped	
3 cloves garlic, minced	
	5 Serve the turkey meatballs over the whole-grain rice.

Per serving: Calories 384 (From Fat 144); Fat 16g (Saturated 3g); Cholesterol 90mg; Sodium 923mg; Carbohydrate 38g (Dietary Fiber 2g); Protein 21g

Preparing Vegetarian Entrees that Pop

Meat and meat products don't have to be present for good, hearty meals fit for entertaining. Putting together the right combination of vegetables, legumes, tofu, and pasta or dumplings can create a meal fit for a king — or you and some friends and family. Adding a complement of herbs and spices gives each dish an anti-inflammatory boost to get your body feeling better.

Yellow Thai Curry with Vegetables and Tofu

Prep time: 15 min • **Cook time:** 10–15 min • **Yield:** 4 servings

Ingredients	Directions
1 cup coconut milk	*1* Bring the coconut milk and vegetable stock to a boil in a medium saucepan. Add the sweet potatoes, and then reduce the heat and simmer, covered, for 10 minutes.
1 cup vegetable broth	
1 cup peeled, chopped sweet potatoes	
3 cloves garlic, minced	*2* Add the garlic, ginger, turmeric, curry powder, cayenne pepper, tofu, broccoli, and mushrooms. Simmer, covered, for 5 to 10 minutes or until the sweet potatoes are easily pierced with a fork and the broccoli is tender but still slightly crisp.
1 tablespoon fresh, grated ginger	
1 teaspoon turmeric	
2 teaspoons curry powder	
½ teaspoon red cayenne pepper	*3* Serve the curry over brown rice and top with the scallions.
2 cups firm tofu, cut into cubes	
1 cup broccoli	
1 cup mushrooms, sliced	
2 cups cooked brown rice	
1 scallion, diced	

Per serving: Calories 464 (From Fat 210); Fat 23g (Saturated 12g); Cholesterol 0mg; Sodium 156mg; Carbohydrate 46g (Dietary Fiber 8g); Protein 24g

Steamed Vegetable Dumplings

Prep time: 30 min • **Cook time:** 1 hr • **Yield:** 7 servings

Ingredients	*Directions*
2 scallions, chopped	*1* In a medium bowl, combine the scallions, ginger, garlic, bean sprouts, mushrooms, hoisin sauce, tamari sauce, and sesame oil. Add the tofu to the sauce mixture and stir to coat the tofu.
1 tablespoon fresh minced ginger	
1 tablespoon minced garlic	
½ cup bean sprouts	*2* Remove the wonton wrappers from the package and keep them under a damp cloth until you need them. Working with one wrapper at a time, lightly brush the edges with water before placing a teaspoon of the tofu mixture in the middle.
½ cup mushrooms, sliced	
1 tablespoon sugar-free, wheat-free hoisin or Peking sauce	
1 tablespoon wheat-free tamari sauce	*3* Take one corner of the wonton and fold it diagonally over the tofu mixture, forming a triangle. Press the edges of the wrapper together to close the dumpling.
1 tablespoon sesame oil	
½ pound firm tofu, cut into 1-inch pieces	*4* After filling all the wrappers, bring ½ inch of water to a simmer in a pot with a steamer basket. Steam the dumplings in batches, covered, for 10 to 15 minutes over medium heat. Transfer the cooked dumplings to a large bowl and cover with plastic wrap until all the dumplings are done. Add more water to the pot in between batches for steaming.
35 wonton wrappers	
2 tablespoons chopped fresh cilantro	
	5 Serve with a sprinkling of cilantro.

Per serving: Calories 197 (From Fat 49); Fat 6g (Saturated 1g); Cholesterol 4mg; Sodium 373mg; Carbohydrate 28g (Dietary Fiber 3g); Protein 10g

Tip: If you have a bamboo steamer basket, line the bottom with lettuce or cabbage leaves or parchment paper to prevent the dumplings from sticking. You should be able to steam eight dumplings at a time in a bamboo steamer. If you don't have a bamboo steamer, you can use a collapsible metal steamer; brush the bottom with a little sesame oil to prevent sticking.

Vegetarian Poppy Seed Burgers

Prep time: 30 min • **Cook time:** 1 hr • **Yield:** 4 servings

Ingredients	Directions
1 cup dried yellow split peas 2½ cups water 4 tablespoons extra-virgin olive oil, divided 1 onion, chopped 1 clove garlic, chopped 1 cup mushrooms, finely chopped 2 tablespoons sunflower seeds, without shells 2 tablespoons sesame seeds 1 tablespoon poppy seeds ¼ cup chopped fresh cilantro 1 teaspoon ground cumin 2 eggs ¼ cup ground flaxseed 2 cups arugula or mixed greens 2½ tablespoons brewer's yeast or nutritional yeast (optional)	**1** Rinse the yellow split peas and drain them. Place the peas in a saucepan with the water. Bring the water to a boil over medium-high heat; then reduce the heat and simmer for 30 to 40 minutes or until the peas are cooked and have absorbed the water. **2** Heat 2 tablespoons of the olive oil in a skillet over medium heat. Sauté the garlic, onion, and mushrooms for 2 to 5 minutes or until they're soft. **3** Crush the sunflower seeds. Combine the cooked split peas, mushroom mixture, sunflower seeds, sesame seeds, poppy seeds, cilantro, cumin, wheat germ, and eggs. Mix to form a soft dough. **4** Form the mixture into eight balls and then flatten them into small patties. **5** Heat the remaining 2 tablespoons olive oil in a large skillet over medium heat. Cook the patties in batches until they're slightly crispy but not burned, about 7 to 9 minutes, flipping the patties halfway through the cooking time. **6** Serve the burgers on a bed of arugula or mixed greens. Sprinkle each burger with 1 teaspoon brewer's yeast (if desired).

Per serving: Calories 407 (From Fat 200); Fat 22g (Saturated 3g); Cholesterol 106mg; Sodium 43mg; Carbohydrate 37g (Dietary Fiber 14g); Protein 19g

Note: Brewer's yeast has many health benefits, including acting as a digestive aid. It's high in B vitamins as well as the antioxidants chromium and selenium. It's also high in protein. You can find brewer's yeast at your local health food store or at many drugstores. Avoid brewer's yeast if you're susceptible to vaginal yeast infections.

Chapter 15

Topping It Off: Desserts

Go ahead, take that slice of cheesecake. Or grab a chocolate truffle. How about a passion fruit smoothie? Sounds too good to be true, doesn't it? You're making the switch to an anti-inflammatory lifestyle, changing out your pantry and introducing new things into your diet. Now we're talking *desserts?*

As with anything else, desserts are fine in moderation, and these recipes make them even better yet. Here we use applesauce or natural sweeteners like agave nectar, honey, or stevia in place of sugar, taking much of the inflammatory properties out of each item. So go ahead, grab that cookie. Enjoy your desserts without worrying about the inflammation they won't be causing.

Refreshing Desserts: Smoothies, Parfaits, and More

There's nothing more refreshing than a crisp, cold smoothie or a creamy parfait, particularly if it's filled with fresh fruit bursting with flavor. But even the healthiest desserts need to be eaten in moderation, making portion control just as important with these desserts and sweet treats as it is with anything else you eat.

Overindulgence may seem too easy — a larger parfait glass, eating more than one popsicle, using a large bowl instead of a smaller one — but keep in mind the nutritional values offered in these recipes, as well as the anti-inflammatory benefits, are for the number of servings listed. Despite their anti-inflammatory properties, these desserts can actually work against you if you take too much.

Passion Fruit Smoothie

Prep time: 15 min • **Cook time:** None • **Yield:** 4 servings

Ingredients	Directions
2 passion fruits, peeled, seeded, and cut into small pieces, or 2–3 tablespoons passion fruit puree	*1* Put the passion fruit, banana, blueberries, rose water, and lemon juice in a blender and blend until smooth.
1 ripe banana, peeled and sliced	*2* To the blender, add the yogurt or milk, honey, and cinnamon and blend for 5 to 10 seconds longer. Pour into glasses to serve.
1 cup fresh blueberries	
1 teaspoon rose water	
2 tablespoons fresh lemon juice	
1 cup plain Greek yogurt, 0–2% fat, or dairy-free milk	
2 teaspoons raw, unprocessed honey	
1 teaspoon cinnamon	

Per serving: Calories 108 (From Fat 12); Fat 1g (Saturated 1g); Cholesterol 4mg; Sodium 21mg; Carbohydrate 21g (Dietary Fiber 3g); Protein 6g

Note: You can find rose water in many gourmet food stores or on specialty websites, such as www.olivenation.com.

Tip: If your smoothie is too thick for your preference, add an extra splash or two of lemon juice and blend for just a few more seconds.

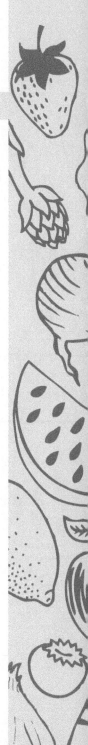

Berry Cherry Popsicles

Prep time: 1 hr, 30 min • **Cook time:** None • **Yield:** 6 servings

Ingredients	Directions
1 cup fresh blueberries	*1* Combine the blueberries, raspberries, cherries, almond milk, and agave nectar in a blender and blend until smooth.
1 cup fresh raspberries	
1 cup fresh cherries, pits and stems removed	
½ cup almond milk	*2* Pour about a half cup of the mixture into each of 6 paper cups. Set the cups on a tray and place the tray in the freezer for about 20 minutes. Remove the tray and place a popsicle stick or plastic spoon in the center of each cup, spoon-side down.
2 tablespoons agave nectar	
	3 Return the tray to the freezer for at least 1 hour or until the popsicles are completely frozen. To serve, peel away the paper cup.

Per serving: Calories 64 (From Fat 5); Fat 1g (Saturated 0g); Cholesterol 0mg; Sodium 14mg; Carbohydrate 16g (Dietary Fiber 3g); Protein 1g

Strawberry Banana Frozen Yogurt

Prep time: 1 hr • **Cook time:** 3–5 min • **Yield:** 4 servings

Ingredients	*Directions*
¼ cup rice milk 2 tablespoons raw, unprocessed honey	*1* Heat the rice milk in a saucepan over low heat, stirring until it's warmed through. Turn off the heat and stir in the honey.
2 ripe bananas, peeled and sliced 1 cup sliced fresh strawberries ½ cup plain Greek yogurt, 0–2% fat	*2* Combine the bananas, strawberries, and yogurt in a blender and blend until smooth. Divide the mixture among six plastic cups. Place a plastic spoon in the center of each cup.
	3 Freeze the yogurt cups for 1 hour or overnight, until the yogurt is frozen. Squeeze out the frozen yogurt from each cup or eat it with the plastic spoon as it softens.

Per serving: Calories 122 (From Fat 2); Fat 0g (Saturated 0g); Cholesterol 0mg; Sodium 17mg; Carbohydrate 29g (Dietary Fiber 3g); Protein 3g

Note: Dairy products don't work for everyone on an anti-inflammatory diet. If you have dairy sensitivities or lactose intolerance, substitute soy or coconut products instead.

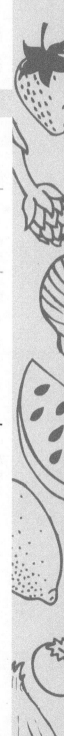

Fruit and Yogurt Parfait with Chocolate and Almonds

Prep time: 15 min • **Cook time:** 5–10 min • **Yield:** 4 servings

Ingredients	*Directions*
½ cup fresh blueberries (or fruit of choice)	*1* Combine the blueberries, honey, and almond extract in a small bowl, and mix well.
4 tablespoons raw, unprocessed honey	
1 teaspoon pure almond extract	*2* Place ½ cup yogurt in each of four serving dishes. Top the yogurt with equal amounts of the sweetened blueberries.
2 cups dairy-free strawberry yogurt	
3 ounces dark chocolate	*3* Set a metal bowl on top of a simmering saucepan of water. Place the chocolate in the bowl and stir until it's melted.
4 teaspoons slivered almonds	
	4 Drizzle the chocolate over each serving of yogurt and blueberries. Top each serving with 1 teaspoon slivered almonds.

Per serving: Calories 299 (From Fat 76); Fat 8g (Saturated 5g); Cholesterol 0mg; Sodium 15mg; Carbohydrate 53g (Dietary Fiber 3g); Protein 4g

Note: Dairy products don't work for everyone on an anti-inflammatory diet. If you have dairy sensitivities or lactose intolerance, substitute soy or coconut products instead.

Going Traditional with Cookies, Rice Pudding, and Baked Fruit Desserts

Switching to an anti-inflammatory lifestyle and diet doesn't mean having to go without baked goods. The great thing about these desserts is that they combine hearty antioxidant-filled nuts with spices that help curb cancer, fight diabetes, and prevent heart disease. Ginger, used for centuries to aid everything from cancers and morning sickness to migraines and the flu, is a key ingredient in many of these recipes, adding to their healthy benefits. (Figure 15-1 shows you how to prepare and mince ginger.)

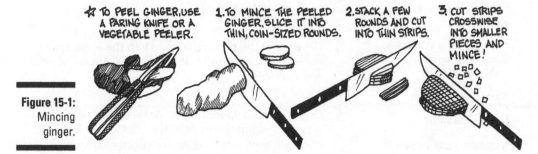

MINCING PEELED GINGER

☆ TO PEEL GINGER, USE A PARING KNIFE OR A VEGETABLE PEELER.

1. TO MINCE THE PEELED GINGER, SLICE IT INTO THIN, COIN-SIZED ROUNDS.

2. STACK A FEW ROUNDS AND CUT INTO THIN STRIPS.

3. CUT STRIPS CROSSWISE INTO SMALLER PIECES AND MINCE!

Figure 15-1:
Mincing ginger.

One of the foundational ingredients in baked goods is flour, and if you have a gluten allergy or sensitivity, gluten-free flours and pastries are an option for you. Some gluten-free flours suitable for baking are rice flour, chickpea flour, sorghum flour, and buckwheat flour. People with gluten intolerance and sensitivity will tolerate oats, which are naturally gluten-free, and most people with celiac disease will be fine with oats as long as they're not produced in a facility that shares equipment with gluten-containing products.

When opting for a cookie for dessert, stick to just one. Don't overindulge in sweet temptation; instead, savor one cookie now and leave yourself an opening to enjoy another one later, if you wish.

Oatmeal Walnut Cookies

Prep time: 20 min • **Cook time:** 10–15 min • **Yield:** 12 servings

Ingredients	Directions
2 tablespoons softened coconut butter, divided	**1** Preheat the oven to 350 degrees. Spread 1 tablespoon of the coconut butter on a baking sheet.
½ cup agave nectar	
¼ cup unsweetened applesauce	**2** Stir together the agave nectar, applesauce, egg, remaining tablespoon of coconut butter, and vanilla extract.
1 egg	
1 teaspoon pure vanilla extract	**3** In a separate bowl, combine the oats, flour, salt, baking powder, and cinnamon.
1 cup certified gluten-free quick-cooking or old-fashioned oats	**4** Gently fold the dry ingredients into the applesauce mixture and stir until just blended. Mix in the walnuts and currants.
¾ cup sorghum flour	
¼ teaspoon salt	**5** Drop rounded spoonfuls of cookie dough onto the greased baking sheet. Bake the cookies for 10 to 12 minutes or until the edges are slightly browned and the centers spring back to the touch.
½ teaspoon baking powder	
1 teaspoon cinnamon	
¼ cup chopped walnuts	
¼ cup dried currants or raisins	

Per serving: Calories 140 (From Fat 38); Fat 4g (Saturated 2g); Cholesterol 18mg; Sodium 71mg; Carbohydrate 24g (Dietary Fiber 3g); Protein 3g

Chocolate Hazelnut Cookies

Prep time: 20 min • **Cook time:** 10–15 min • **Yield:** 16 servings

Ingredients	*Directions*
1 cup plus 1 tablespoon softened coconut butter, divided	*1* Preheat the oven to 350 degrees. Spread 1 tablespoon of the coconut butter on a baking sheet.
½ cup stevia	
1 egg	*2* In a large bowl, blend 1 cup softened coconut butter with the stevia, egg, coconut milk, and vanilla extract.
¼ cup coconut milk	
1 teaspoon pure vanilla extract	
4 cups unbleached white flour	*3* In a separate bowl, combine the flour, baking powder, cardamom, and salt.
2 teaspoons baking powder	
½ teaspoon ground cardamom seeds	*4* Gently fold the dry ingredients into the butter mixture and stir until just blended. Mix in the hazelnuts and cocoa nibs.
½ teaspoon salt	
¼ cup roasted hazelnuts, roughly chopped	*5* Drop rounded spoonfuls of cookie dough onto the greased baking sheet. Bake the cookies for 10 to 12 minutes or until the edges are slightly browned and the centers spring back to the touch.
¼ cup cocoa nibs	

Per serving: Calories 255 (From Fat 122); Fat 14g (Saturated 10g); Cholesterol 13mg; Sodium 131mg; Carbohydrate 29g (Dietary Fiber 4g); Protein 5g

Note: Cocoa nibs are roasted cocoa beans separated from their husks and broken into bits. They're available at many gourmet food stores.

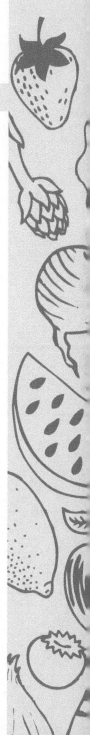

Rice Pudding with Pomegranate Seeds

Prep time: 15 min • **Cook time:** 30–40 min • **Yield:** 4 servings

Ingredients	*Directions*
1 cup basmati rice	*1* Rinse and drain the rice.
1 cup water	
1 cup coconut milk	*2* Put the rice into a saucepan. Add the water, coconut milk, cardamom, and 1 tablespoon of the cinnamon.
2 tablespoons ground cardamom seeds	
2 tablespoons cinnamon, divided	*3* Bring the mixture to a boil over medium heat. Reduce the heat and cook the rice, covered, for 30 to 40 minutes or until the rice is tender.
½ cup chopped walnuts	
1 whole pomegranate, deseeded	*4* Divide the rice pudding into four bowls. Top each bowl with 2 tablespoons chopped walnuts, 1 to 2 tablespoons pomegranate seeds, and a dash of cinnamon or to taste.

Per serving: Calories 444 (From Fat 204); Fat 23g (Saturated 12g); Cholesterol 0mg; Sodium 10mg; Carbohydrate 62g (Dietary Fiber 7g); Protein 7g

Tip: To easily and more cleanly deseed the pomegranate, cut the crown from the fruit and quarter the flesh, being careful not to puncture the seeds. Immerse the pomegranate in a bowl of water and carefully separate the fruit at the perforations. With your hands still in the water, separate the seeds from the membrane and the flesh.

Baked Apples with Walnuts and Cinnamon

Prep time: 10 min • **Cook time:** 20–30 min • **Yield:** 6 servings

Ingredients	Directions
½ cup chopped walnuts 2 tablespoons chopped dates 1½ cups certified gluten-free quick-cooking oats 1 tablespoon cinnamon ½ teaspoon nutmeg 1 teaspoon pure vanilla extract ¼ cup maple syrup 4 apples, peeled, cored, and sliced	**1** Preheat the oven to 300 degrees. Sprinkle a glass baking dish with a little water and then line it with parchment paper cut to fit the bottom of the dish. **2** Combine the walnuts, dates, oats, cinnamon, nutmeg, vanilla, and maple syrup in a small bowl. **3** Place the apple slices in the bottom of the lined baking dish. Top the apples with the oatmeal mixture. **4** Bake for 20 to 30 minutes or until the apples are soft.

Per serving: Calories 224 (From Fat 65); Fat 7g (Saturated 1g); Cholesterol 0mg; Sodium 2mg; Carbohydrate 38g (Dietary Fiber 5g); Protein 5g

Tip: Some of the best apple varieties for baking include Jonathan, Jonagold, Honeycrisp, and Granny Smith, all of which have a crisp, tart flavor and firmer flesh that hold up well to baking.

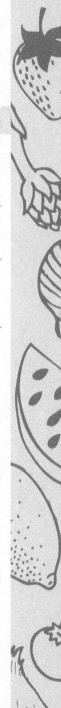

Baked Pears with Ginger Syrup

Prep time: 15 min • **Cook time:** 10–15 min • **Yield:** 4 servings

Ingredients	Directions
4 firm pears, peeled, cored, and sliced in half 2 tablespoons raw, unprocessed honey 2 tablespoons ginger syrup (see the following recipe) 1 teaspoon cinnamon	**1** Preheat the oven to 375 degrees. Sprinkle a glass baking dish with a little water and then line it with parchment paper cut to fit the bottom of the dish. **2** Place the pear halves, cut side down, in the bottom of the lined baking dish. Bake the pears for 10 to 15 minutes or until they're softened. **3** While the pears bake, combine the honey and ginger syrup. **4** Place two halves of the cooked pears on each plate. Spoon 1 to 2 tablespoons of the syrup mixture onto each half and sprinkle the pears with cinnamon.

Ginger Syrup

Ingredients	Directions
1-inch piece fresh ginger ½ cup water 2 tablespoons raw, unprocessed honey	**1** Peel and thinly slice the piece of fresh ginger. **2** Place the ginger, water, and honey in a small saucepan. Simmer on medium-low heat for 15 minutes or until it thickens to the consistency of syrup.

Per serving: Calories 114 (From Fat 1); Fat 0g (Saturated 0g); Cholesterol 0mg; Sodium 7mg; Carbohydrate 28g (Dietary Fiber 1g); Protein 1g

Tip: You can store any unused ginger syrup in the refrigerator for a few days. Drizzle it over fresh fruit, use it on toast like you would honey, or mix it in with granola for added flavor.

Satisfying Your Craving for Chocolate

Oh yes, we said *chocolate*. What dessert chapter would be complete without a section with chocolate? You've probably heard all the bad things people say about chocolate: It's bad for your skin, it has too much sugar, and it's not good for you.

Truth is, they're wrong. About all of it. Chocolate, in particular dark chocolate, is full of healthy antioxidants and *polyphenols* — the antioxidants found in white and green tea that protect against heart disease by inhibiting the oxidation of LDL, or bad cholesterol.

In addition to chocolate, these recipes use coconut butter. Like human breast milk, coconut butter is rich in lauric acid and works to build immunity and protect against bad bacteria and viruses. You can find it in gourmet or specialty food stores as well as many health food stores.

These recipes call for the use of a double boiler, which is a specialized piece of cooking equipment usually containing two sizes of saucepans, with one fitting on top of the other. The bottom pan holds water for boiling and the top pan is used for melting chocolate or making candy. If you don't have or don't want to purchase a dedicated double boiler, you can create your own using a small saucepan and a metal bowl that sits on top but doesn't rest on the bottom of the saucepan. Put some water in the saucepan to simmer, and it will heat up the metal bowl, allowing you to melt chocolate.

Chocolate-Covered Fresh Fruit

Prep time: 10 min • **Cook time:** 5 min • **Yield:** 12 servings

Ingredients	*Directions*
16 ounces dark chocolate, roughly chopped	*1* Line a baking sheet with parchment paper. Melt the dark chocolate, coconut butter, and honey in a double boiler over low heat, stirring until the chocolate is melted. Stir in the vanilla extract.
2 tablespoons softened coconut butter	
2 tablespoons raw, unprocessed honey	*2* Dip the fruit in the chocolate mixture and place it on the parchment. Refrigerate the dipped fruit for 10 to 15 minutes before serving.
1 teaspoon pure vanilla extract	
12 servings cut fresh fruit, washed and dried (strawberries, melon bites, orange slices, and other favorites)	

Per serving: Calories 275 (From Fat 130); Fat 15g (Saturated 9g); Cholesterol 0mg; Sodium 2mg; Carbohydrate 36g (Dietary Fiber 7g); Protein 3g

Chocolate-Covered Ginger Bites

Prep time: 10 min • **Cook time:** 5 min • **Yield:** 3 servings

Ingredients	*Directions*
Six 1-inch slices candied or crystallized ginger **½ cup chopped dark chocolate**	*1* Line a baking sheet with parchment paper. Melt the dark chocolate in a double boiler over low heat, stirring until the chocolate is melted.
1 tablespoon crushed walnuts	*2* Dip the ginger pieces in the melted chocolate and place them on the parchment. Sprinkle the ginger pieces with crushed walnuts. Refrigerate for 5 minutes before serving.

Per serving: *Calories 192 (From Fat 99); Fat 11g (Saturated 6g); Cholesterol 0mg; Sodium 2mg; Carbohydrate 23g (Dietary Fiber 2g); Protein 2g*

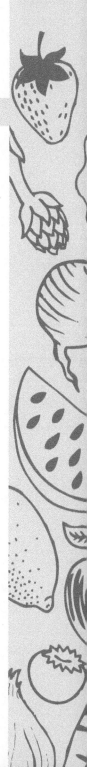

Part IV
Living an Anti-Inflammatory Lifestyle

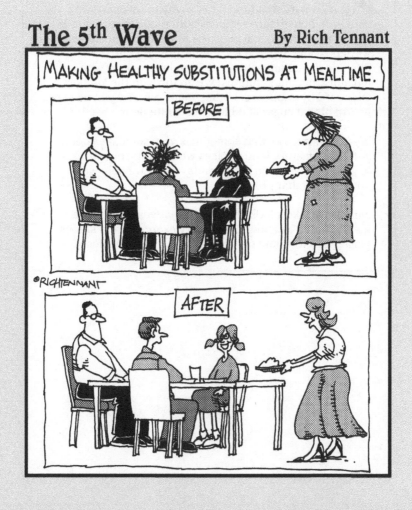

The 5th Wave   By Rich Tennant

MAKING HEALTHY SUBSTITUTIONS AT MEALTIME.

BEFORE

AFTER

In this part . . .

*J*ust as food can trigger inflammation, so can the way
you prepare that food. That's why in this part, we
show you how to take recipes (both those we provide in
Part III and others) and cook the foods in the healthiest
ways possible. We also walk you through your kitchen,
ditching the inflammatory foods and restocking with anti-
inflammatory substitutions. We go through the kitchen
cupboard by cupboard, letting you know why you need to
get rid of that sugar and bleached white flour.

We recognize, too, that sometimes you can make good,
anti-inflammatory food choices when eating out —
including at fast-food restaurants — and we help walk
you through that process.

Finally, we take a look at drug alternatives and supplements as well as anti-inflammatory exercises and simple
yoga poses to round out the anti-inflammatory lifestyle.

Chapter 16

Making Home Cooking Less Inflammatory

In This Chapter

▶ Getting rid of the inflammatory foods and filling up the kitchen right

▶ Using the best cooking methods

▶ Experimenting with healthier ways to prepare food

*T*he best menu for anti-inflammatory foods is one you create at home when you're aware of all ingredients and can use all fresh, local, seasonal, and organic products. When you're in control of ingredients and how they're cooked, you know exactly what you're eating. To do that in the best way possible, however, you have to make sure your kitchen is ready.

Take a good look around your kitchen: Open the cupboard doors, swing around the Lazy Susan, even take a peek inside your spice cabinet and refrigerator. Chances are pretty good you're playing host to a lot of inflammatory foods. Some inflammatory ingredients may even be hidden, such as artificial sweeteners in baby foods, monosodium glutamate (MSG) in chicken broth, or even hydrogenated fats in so-called "health food" bars.

Making the switch to an anti-inflammatory lifestyle means making changes — starting right in your kitchen. Revamping the ingredients in your kitchen also makes it easier to keep to an anti-inflammatory diet on the fly. From the kinds of cereals and baking supplies you have on hand down to how you prepare the foods you eat, this chapter takes you through the home-cooking modifications that can keep you healthy and inflammation-free.

Stocking an Anti-Inflammatory Kitchen

When you're considering what to put into your kitchen, you also have to evaluate what you need to take out. Standing in your kitchen doorway thinking about what you need to throw out can seem pretty daunting. Taking it one step — or one category — at a time makes the job much more manageable, so that's the approach we take in the following sections. After you clear out the bad foods from your kitchen, we help you fill it back up the right way.

When you're evaluating what stays and what goes, check out both the nutrition labels and the ingredients lists:

- ✔ **Nutrition label:** Some key things to look for on food labels are the amount of sugars, trans/hydrogenated fat, saturated fat, and total carbohydrates. On a regular diet, the United States Department of Agriculture's recommended amount of sugar is no more than 40 grams, or 10 teaspoons, a day. That sounds like a lot until you look at it this way: Even one small orange has 12 grams of sugar, almost a third of a full day's supply.

- ✔ **Ingredients:** Read all the ingredients so you don't get fooled into thinking something is healthy when it's really filled with inflammatory ingredients. If you just look on the label for the amount of sugars, fats, and carbohydrates, you may miss the MSG, additives, preservatives, and gluten.

Know which foods you need before you go to the store, and know how long it will last before you bring too much of it home. Get in the habit of creating a weekly menu before you go shopping. Make a list of anti-inflammatory entrees and find complementary sides to accompany them. Keep an eye out for healthy alternatives, or ask the people at your local market what some options may be. As with any diet change, the key to success is proper planning.

Flour, sugar, and other baking supplies

Whether a gourmet baker or someone who just makes the occasional batch of cookies, most everyone has some baking ingredients on hand. Flour, sugar, brown sugar, powdered sugar, shortening, vanilla — you know it's in there somewhere. When you find it, toss it. Well, most of it. In the following sections, we tell you what to do with flours, sweeteners, extracts and spices, and the like.

Flours and other starchy things

Start by throwing out the white flour (or at least relegating it to non-food uses, like papier-mâché paste). White flour is refined, which means any nutrients were removed in processing. It can also be a source of inflammation in people with celiac disease or sensitivity to gluten and wheat.

Small changes can make a big difference

It may seem almost too good to be true, but small changes in your diet really can make a big change in your health. Over the years in my practice I (coauthor Artemis) have seen patients reduce their cholesterol from very high levels to normal levels with simple dietary changes: switching from canola or vegetable oil to olive oil for cooking and sautéing, adding in a wider variety and one or two more daily servings of vegetables, and avoiding fried and processed foods. By sharing tips, suggestions, and recipes throughout this book, we've given you a good start in making those very changes and getting on your way to a healthier lifestyle.

By putting a little bit of effort into reading labels, cutting artificial ingredients out of your diet can also have a huge impact on your health. For example, artificial ingredients such as MSG and artificial colors trigger migraine headaches for many people. By avoiding artificial ingredients, many patients have reported an end to years of suffering from migraine headaches.

Artificial ingredients and processed foods are among the factors that contribute to ill health and yet are some of the easiest to change and remove from your lifestyle, simply by reading labels and choosing fresh, natural foods. The benefit to your health, in addition to the reduction of annoying symptoms like headaches and fatigue, is ridding your body of low-level causes of inflammation and preventing the chronic disease that is caused by inflammation.

In addition to eating more vegetables, whole grains, good fats, and lean proteins, taking steps to manage food allergies, sensitivities, and intolerances can have a dramatic impact on your health and can lower levels of inflammation in the body. Many of my patients with autoimmune diseases, such as multiple sclerosis, rheumatoid arthritis, psoriatic arthritis, and Hashimoto's thyroiditis have an allergy or sensitivity to gluten-containing products. By removing gluten from their diets they've been able to reduce their pain and inflammation levels and have an easier time maintaining a normal body weight; plus, many haven't needed to take pharmaceutical medications for their conditions and are instead following an anti-inflammatory diet with great results. Autoimmune diseases will also respond well to an individualized anti-inflammatory diet that your naturopathic physician can work out with you that includes discovering food allergies, sensitivities, and intolerances, and you can work with your rheumatologist to get you feeling the best you can.

Base the type of flour you choose on the types of grains that cause inflammation for you on an individual basis. People with celiac disease or gluten intolerance should avoid wheat, barley, and rye, and most people should avoid corn because it's usually genetically modified. The safest flours for all to use are rice flours, bean flours (such as garbanzo/chickpea), buckwheat flour, quinoa, and millet. Other alternatives deemed safe for people with celiac disease include acorn flour, almond flour, arrowroot, buckwheat, chickpea (chana) flour, and flax. All flours can be stored in airtight containers in the pantry.

Make sure you toss the starchy things too, such as cornstarch. As with flour, it's been refined and stripped of its nutrients. The less pure or original a food is, the more likely it is to contribute to inflammation.

Sweeteners

Toss the white sugar and powdered sugar, which are both refined. Those artificial sweeteners you have sitting next to the sugar? They have to go, too. They're even worse than refined sugars; instead of having the nutrients taken out, these artificial sweeteners have chemicals and preservatives and sometimes even pesticides added in. And not only is corn syrup filled with sugars, but it also has a high amount of preservatives.

In general, go for natural sweeteners that are lower in the glycemic index, such as stevia, agave nectar, raw honey, and rice syrup — and still use them in moderation. For baking purposes, natural unsweetened applesauce, agave nectar, brown rice syrup, stevia, or organic honey can take the place of sugar in almost any recipe. Different natural sweeteners work better in some situations than others, so we discuss substitutions later in "Staying sweet."

Extracts and spices

That bottle of vanilla may not even have any real vanilla bean extract, so be sure to look for pure vanilla extract made from all natural ingredients.

Remember the spice rack, too, and replace the old ones. Many herbs and spices have anti-inflammatory properties, but they lose their nutritional value over time. Want to know if your spices are still good? Put it to your nose; if it's lost color and odor, it's also lost much of its value.

Fats and cooking oils

Knowing the difference between good and bad fats (see Chapter 5) and remembering to choose the right one puts you on the right track for eliminating bad fats from your diet. When looking at cooking oils and solid fats such as butter and margarine, keep saturated fats to a minimum and avoid trans fats altogether. Saturated fats are allowed in small amounts — although most saturated fats increase bad cholesterol, studies haven't shown them to affect good cholesterol (an exception is coconut oil, which helps maintain good cholesterol levels). Trans fats both increase bad cholesterol and decrease good cholesterol, so they're doubly harmful.

Be careful when reading labels — something that reads "0 g trans fat" may actually have up to 0.5 grams in each serving, which means you're not really getting zero trans fats. With a daily recommendation of no more than 2 grams of trans fat, it'd take just four "0 trans fats" items to hit your limit.

Choosing cooking oils

That bottle of good ol' corn oil may have been what you grew up with, but it shouldn't be what you grow old with. There weren't a lot of oil choices for many years. Now, though, you can find different oils for different palates, even for different dishes.

So which oils should you avoid? Skip the palm oil and palm kernel oil, which are full of saturated fats. Vegetable oil is a definite no-no, as are corn oil, safflower oil and sunflower oil (except the high-oleic kinds), soy oil, and cottonseed oil. They all contain very high levels of omega-6 fatty acids, which can contribute to the development of cancers and heart disease, especially if used in higher amounts than anti-inflammatory fats, such as omega-3s.

On the other hand, some oils have some health benefits. Oils with mono-unsaturated or polyunsaturated fats help lower total cholesterol and, more specifically, the LDL cholesterol, which is the real troublemaker. Oils with monounsaturated fats also help to raise the levels of HDL cholesterol — the good one. Here's a list of good cooking oils:

- ✔ Extra-virgin olive oil (use only for short periods and not higher than medium heat)
- ✔ High-oleic safflower oil
- ✔ High-oleic sunflower oil
- ✔ Walnut oil (medium heat only)
- ✔ Avocado oil
- ✔ Grapeseed oil (medium heat only)

For info on the benefits of specific types of cooking oil, see Chapter 5.

Considering solid fats

By definition, *solid fats* are those that are solid at room temperature — shortening, lard, and butter, for example. They come mostly from animal foods but can be made from vegetable oils through hydrogenation. A general rule of thumb when it comes to solid fats is "stay away." Most solid fats are high in saturated fats and/or trans fats and are usually high in cholesterol.

Shortening contains hydrogenated fats that increase bad cholesterol and decrease good cholesterol. Take one look at that vat of spreadable fat, and you just *know* that isn't going to be good for you. Just 1 cup of shortening has more than 2.5 times the amount of fat a person should have in an entire day, raising the red flag on the inflammation charts and increasing your risk of heart disease.

Butter is high in saturated fat. Margarine is generally better than butter — margarine is made from vegetable oils, so it has no cholesterol and is usually high in the good fats. Unfortunately, not all margarines are the same, and some are actually worse for you than butter because they contain trans fats.

The "better" margarine is somewhat spreadable, even from a refrigerated stick. The more solid the margarine, the more trans fat it contains to make it that way.

Dry goods

Beyond the baking supplies and oils in your pantry are the boxed foods: cereals, crackers, pasta, and the like. Unless you've already taken the step to stick with whole grains and sugar-free, toss these boxed goods. If you have celiac disease or gluten sensitivities or allergies, anything with wheat, barley, or rye also needs to go. (*Note:* An allergy elimination diet or blood test can help determine whether you have allergies or sensitivities to wheat or gluten — see Chapter 2. Because wheat or gluten is in so many products, it can become a source of inflammation even if you're not having any major symptoms.)

Traditional pastas and most crackers are made with refined grains, putting them high on the list of foods to avoid in an anti-inflammatory lifestyle. They're also full of starches that quickly break down into sugars. Similarly, many breakfast cereals are filled with sugars and refined flours. Even instant oatmeal, the little flavored packets prepackaged for single servings, are filled with sugars and preservatives. All these highly refined foods may contribute to obesity, diabetes, cardiac issues, and cancer.

However, switching to an anti-inflammatory diet doesn't mean giving up on all the things you love. With breads and cereals, for example, making the switch to whole-grain rather than white, corn, or enriched may be all the change you need. You can keep the plain, old-fashioned or steel-cut oats without all the sugars and artificial flavors. For people who can't eat gluten, any cereals kept on-hand should be wheat-free as well.

Pasta comes in a variety of forms, including brown rice and buckwheat. Either of these options is a good choice over enriched pasta because they both add more vitamins and minerals as well as natural fiber to your diet. Or try some gluten-free varieties of pasta made out of brown rice, quinoa, or chickpea flour. Expect the other pastas to have a unique taste that's different from gluten-containing pastas.

Subscribing to fresh, local produce

Want to try a variety of fresh, local fruits and vegetables at the peak of their ripeness? Many farms offer *Consumer Supported Agriculture (CSA)* programs, which allow consumers to basically subscribe to their produce for a given season. For a set cost, typically an annual premium, consumers get a weekly share of the bounty, usually whatever ripens that week.

When you pick up your box of produce, you can usually trade away anything you don't want.

A large number of the participating farms are organic or are on the way to being certified. To find a CSA near you — or to search for farmers' markets, food co-ops, and other local food sources — check out www.local harvest.org.

Here are some tips on reading nutrition labels of dry goods:

✔ **Flours:** Make sure you look at the types of flours used, and pay attention to the order they're listed in. If enriched flour is listed before the grains, you may be getting the nutritional value of a piece of white bread with a few grains tossed in. Also watch out for foods that name whole-grain flour first but list enriched flours as the second and third ingredients — together, the enriched flours may total more than the whole-grain.

✔ **Sugars:** Look at the sugar content. Something may be advertised as having an increased amount of fiber or less fat but come with an increased amount of sugar or sweetener, too.

Want to know just how much sugar you're getting? Divide the sugar content on the nutrition label by 4 — that's the number of teaspoons of sugar you're getting *per serving*. You want fewer than 10 teaspoons of sugar per day.

Canned foods

Commercially canned food is typically meant to last a long time. The problem is that the can isn't what makes the food inside last so long; it's the countless additives and preservatives that are mixed in with the contents. Some toxic chemicals, such as BPA (bisphenol A), may even leach from the can to the product inside.

Most canned soups and prepared meals have very high levels of sodium, which may lead to high blood pressure, arthritis, and even some colon diseases. Some may even have monosodium glutamate (MSG), a flavor enhancer that has been linked to headaches, heart palpitations, and chest pains. If a food is available another way — fresh, frozen, or dried — go that route before canned.

You can keep jars of pickled foods, like pickles or artichoke hearts, and hand-canned vegetables.

Refrigerated items

The refrigerator is a real hotbed of inflammatory foods, from the condiments in the door to the meats in the drawer. Many condiments are high in sugar or sugar substitutes, such as high-fructose corn syrup, and therefore follow the lead of other high-sugar foods. Condiments such as soy sauce, teriyaki sauce, and Worcestershire sauce are also very high in sodium. Many soy sauces also contain wheat; if you're sensitive to wheat or gluten, you can substitute wheat-free tamari sauce.

Processed meats, such as sandwich meats, are filled with preservatives and sodium and cancer-causing nitrites, creating an opening for heart disease and obesity. Even the margarine and butter in the fridge are full of the wrong kinds of fats and oils (see the earlier section "Fats and cooking oils").

Some things that are okay to hold onto include yogurts that are 0 to 2 percent milkfat and made with live cultures, as well as Greek yogurt. Most people can tolerate and benefit from fermented dairy products because the nutrients are better absorbed and available through the fermentation process, which eliminates the lactose and allergenic components or makes them less active.

If you can tolerate other dairy products, unpasteurized (raw) forms from organic, grass-fed animals are best because they're higher in nutrients. Try to stick with goat- or sheep-based dairy products over cow's milk products.

Fruits and vegetables

On a scale of 1 to 10 of the best ways to get inflammation-fighting fruits and veggies, buying fresh rates a 15. The fruits and vegetables with the most positive impact on your health are those fresh, organic, locally grown items you find in local markets or, in the right season, at farmers' markets. These foods are much less likely to have been sprayed with pesticides or to have been injected with some form of product enhancer. Buying local, organic vegetables ensures the produce is ripe and free from harmful chemicals.

When buying fresh fruits and vegetables, get just what you think you'll use in a few days' time. Fresh produce doesn't last long, but the benefits of adding it to your diet far outweigh the extra shopping trips.

The next-best option is getting frozen veggies. Although they may still be exposed to some preservatives, the amount of chemicals used is greatly reduced from that in canned vegetables. Before being frozen, many of these vegetables are *blanched,* which means they're briefly dipped in boiling water, just enough to cook without the danger of overcooking. That allows them to retain their color and fresh taste.

Fruits and vegetables take quite a beating going from the farm to the can and lose much of their nutritional value in the process. Even those boasting "low sodium" or "packed in natural juices" are exposed to preservatives and other chemicals to make them last longer, and the toxicity in some cans may be leaching into the foods inside. Canned fruits, although they may not have the sodium levels that canned vegetables pose, often have high levels of high-fructose syrup or other sugars. The sugars in those products can help lead to obesity, diabetes, and some cancers.

Beverages

In general, the more natural a beverage is, the better it is for you and your anti-inflammatory lifestyle. Diet sodas are obviously out. The artificial sweeteners in diet sodas provide few calories, but they create bigger problems: In addition to making you crave food, some artificial sweeteners have been linked to headaches and some cancers. Flavored juice drinks are often full of sugars without providing the benefits of fruit.

So after you ditch the soda, the flavored juice drinks, and other "toxic" drinks, what do you replace them with? You can drink plenty of things when you're following an anti-inflammatory diet. White, green, and black teas are fine (see the nearby "The truth about teas" sidebar), and so is the occasional organic soda. The best soda choice is one that's naturally sweetened with stevia, such as Zevia or Blue Sky Soda, which you can find in natural food stores.

Most 100-percent fruit juices are also fine. Keep in mind, though, that even natural fruit juices have an elevated level of natural sugars, so drink those in moderation. Better yet, dilute them with water to decrease the amount of sugar per serving. If you still want that soda-like beverage, dilute the fruit juice with soda water.

The truth about teas

Some herbal teas — chamomile, peppermint, mangosteen — aren't made from actual tea leaves; instead, the herbs are infused when they're steeped in water. They still make great beverages with many medicinal and anti-inflammatory properties.

True teas — those that come from the leaves of a Chinese evergreen — include white tea, black tea, green tea, and oolong. Green tea has long been praised for its healing benefits, but both green tea and black tea have been shown to prevent heart disease and strengthen the immune system. Because white tea is made from immature tea leaves that are left close to their natural state, white tea contains more *polyphenols,* the antioxidant that kills cancer-causing cells, than any other type of tea. Many studies tout the anti-cancer benefits of other teas, too, especially toward gastric, esophageal, and skin cancers.

Making tea from whole leaves is usually better than using teabags, which are typically made from low tea grades. Steeping loose-leaf tea allows room for water to be absorbed and the leaves to expand, emitting the variety of vitamins, minerals, and flavors.

Many people have some level of lactose intolerance, dairy allergies, or dairy sensitivity, so you can replace cow's milk with dairy-free alternatives, such as almond milk, non-GMO (genetically modified organism) soymilk, rice milk, or hemp milk. Also, goat's milk may be better tolerated than cow's milk because goats are generally grass-fed/pastured rather than kept in cow cities (concentrated animal-feeding operations, or CAFOs). If you're one of the rare people who can tolerate cow's milk, opt for milk from organic, grass-fed animals.

Choosing the Right Cooking Methods

Knowing *what* to eat gets you started toward living an anti-inflammatory lifestyle, but unless you know how to prepare the food properly, you can undo all that good you just did. The following sections cover some of the best ways to cook anti-inflammatory foods.

One thing to consider before you get that pan out: Try to make at least half of the food you consume be raw. Raw foods, such as raw vegetables, tend to be higher in vitamins, minerals, fiber, and digestive enzymes than the cooked versions. Here are raw food choices to add to your diet in general:

✔ Raw vegetables and fruits

✔ Sprouted beans, nuts, seeds, and grains

✔ Fresh juices, such as from beets, ginger, and apples (experiment with a juicer and try to have at least one serving of a vegetable-based juice daily)

However, raw foods are not the best option for certain nutrients. Although cooking destroys some nutrients, it increases the *bioavailabilty* of others — in other words, it helps your body better access and use those nutrients. For example, *phytic acid* is a chemical found in raw nuts, seeds, and grains that inhibits absorption of important minerals, such as calcium, magnesium, zinc, and iron. Heating destroys the phytic acid, allowing your body to better absorb and utilize the minerals found in these foods. Therefore, cooking at least half of your foods allows for maximal absorption of these anti-inflammatory and needed minerals.

Baking meats, veggies, and more

Baking isn't just for cakes and cookies; baking meats and poultry as well as seafood, fruits, and vegetables can keep the nutrients in without adding a lot of fat or other inflammatory consequences.

Here are a few baking tips:

✔ Put your meat or poultry, veggies, or fruit in the center of a good baking dish, preferably glass or ceramic. Be sure to allow enough room around the sides to let hot air circulate.

✔ Put vegetables on the bottom of the baking dish with the meat or fish on top. This adds natural moisture to the baking pan and lets the juices seep into the vegetables and create added flavor.

✔ Add water or liquids to the baking pan. Heating meat proteins can lead to inflammatory advanced glycation end-products (AGE) — the dark brown or burnt places you can get from high-heat cooking, such as when grilling. The chemical reaction can't occur as readily in the presence of water. For some meats and poultry, feel free to add a bit of a low-sodium homemade marinade before covering.

✔ Want to keep the moisture in without adding unnecessary fats? Put a cover on the baking dish, whether you're using a lid or simply folding aluminum foil around the top and cinching the edges. Or try baking with parchment paper. Using the paper as an envelope or packet for your food — whether it's just veggies or those perfectly seasoned salmon steaks — can help the food cook with steam while retaining its natural juices.

Steaming things up

One of the easiest ways to cook food is to steam it, usually by putting the food — whether it's meat or seafood, fruits or vegetables, beans or legumes — in a slotted basket over a pan of water and then covering the pan. You can also use a vegetable steamer, rice cooker, or bamboo steamer for certain foods.

Here are some steaming tips:

✔ **Vegetables:** When steaming vegetables, be sure not to overcook them. Vegetables should retain their natural color — or become even brighter in color — and maintain an amount of crispness and their nutrients. If the fork goes in and then comes out easily, the vegetables are done.

✔ **Fish and seafood:** Cook fish until it flakes but the sides and edges don't start to curl. Shellfish — shrimp, crab, and lobster, for example — is done when it's opaque throughout. Be sure the item is cooked through, but don't overcook. Overcooking fish and seafood can make it too chewy and take away the anti-inflammatory benefits.

✔ **Herbs and spices:** Using certain herbs and spices while steaming infuses the flavor into the food, further enhancing the taste without depleting any of the nutrients. Add dried herbs, such as rosemary and sage, while food is simmering or in marinades. Add root-based spices, such as ginger and turmeric, while the food is steaming. Most green herbs are best added at the end of the cooking to retain their flavor and antioxidant properties, so add fresh parsley, mint, and dill at the end of cooking.

Poaching delicate foods

Poaching is a good lowfat way to cook your meat because you don't add additional fats, such as oils, when you're cooking. The flavor remains strong, depending on the herbs and spices you use, because as the meat's own liquids cook off, the herbs and spices mix with the poaching liquid and become infused back into the meat.

Poaching is a lot like steaming without the basket: Put enough of your poaching liquid — whether it's water, light marinade, or a low-sodium, MSG-free stock — in the bottom of a pan, making sure you have enough to completely cover the food by about an inch. Bring the liquid to a boil and add your meat or seafood (or even vegetables). Reduce the heat to the right temperature for the meat: For fish it's between 175 degrees and 185 degrees, and for chicken and beef it's between 160 degrees and 175 degrees.

Don't worry if you don't have a thermometer; keep the water just below a simmer, with the water rippling but not bubbling. Cook according to the size of the meat or fish: An 8-ounce piece of fish takes about 10 minutes, and chicken and beef of the same size take about twice as long.

When your meat is done cooking, don't toss the liquid. Instead, throw in a few vegetables and make it into a soup for later meals.

Healthy frying methods

Whether you're looking at potatoes or other vegetables, meat, or anything else, fried foods generally aren't good for you. Frying involves excess oils — typically unhealthy oils — as well as batter or other fry blends. If a food requires a substantial amount of fats (oil, lard, and so on) to cook, then chances are it's not healthy at all. The exception to this rule is stir-frying; when done in the proper oil, stir-frying can be a much healthier option.

Unlike foods that are french-fried or deep-fried, stir-fried foods are cooked with a small amount of oil (or none at all) at high temperatures for a very short amount of time. Because the food is cooked so quickly, there's not much of a chance for the food to absorb the oil. What vegetables do retain during stir-frying are their beneficial nutrients; because the foods are exposed to heat for such a short time, the nutrients don't have time to break down.

One thing to keep in mind when cooking with any oil is the oil's *smoke point*. That's the temperature at which the heated oil breaks down and begins to smoke. Different oils have different smoke points, and some oils just aren't meant to be used for frying. The heat changes the properties of the oil and may make an otherwise okay oil inflammatory.

The best oils to use at high temperatures are unrefined oils with high anti-oxidant and anti-inflammatory properties, such as virgin olive oil or coconut oil. Olive oil is good for sautéing over medium heat, so it's often used in Mediterranean cooking.

Other methods: Grilling, broiling, and microwaving

High-temperature grilling or broiling involves dry-cooking the meat and allowing the fats to drip off. However, when excessive temperatures are involved, the fats and proteins in meat turn into *heterocyclic amines* (HAs), which may raise the risk of certain cancers. That doesn't mean you have to toss the grill.

Keep grilling fish and vegetables, which don't need much time on the grill, and when you really have to have that grilled meat, choose chicken, turkey, wild game, and bison.

Generally speaking, cooking your food in a microwave destroys the nutrients in food because it's a high-heat cooking method. We don't advise it on an anti-inflammatory diet.

Making Favorite Dishes Less Inflammatory

The worst part of starting any new diet is giving up unhealthy favorites. But in many cases, an anti-inflammatory diet doesn't mean walking away — as long as you're willing to make a few adjustments. Inflammation can come from food sensitivities, such as to wheat products or dairy; how foods are prepared; or from the foods themselves. A little adjustment here and a substitution there, and you've resurrected your favorite dish.

Using this for that: Healthy substitutions in main dishes and sides

If you don't mind switching things up a bit, you have plenty of ways to make those inflammatory foods work for you rather than against you. Not sure where to start? Here's a list to help you get started:

- **Butter on vegetables:** There's no arguing that butter can make steamed or boiled vegetables taste oh-so-good. A healthier option for those vegetables is to mix some olive oil with a bit of lemon pepper and spray or drizzle on. The lemon pepper can help you skip the salt, too.

- **Breading:** Getting ready to bread some chicken or beef (free-range, not farmed) for baking or steaming? Grind some oatmeal or rice crackers in a food processor or food chopper, enough to make it fine. Add some spices, and you're set. Depending on the recipe, you can also use ground nuts, such as almonds or pine nuts.

- **Potatoes and their fixings:** White potatoes are high in starch and sugars but can be easily replaced with sweet potatoes — even in the mashed variety. Instead of making the mashed potatoes with butter and milk, try a bit of olive oil or plain yogurt with a sprinkle of chives.

Staying sweet

Some recipes are just too difficult to toss aside, and with these sugar substitutes, you may not have to. Here's a list of some of the things you can use in place of traditional sweeteners when baking:

- ✔ **Stevia:** Stevia, a natural sweetener that's safe for diabetics, comes granulated or in liquid form. Use granulated stevia as a substitute for refined sugar in baking, tea, and other hot beverages. Replace 1 cup sugar with 1 teaspoon liquid stevia, ⅓ to ½ teaspoon stevia extract powder, or 18–24 packets of granulate stevia.

- ✔ **Honey:** Use raw, unprocessed honey in tea, hot beverages, and bread-making. Replace half the granulated sugar with honey for a chewier consistency in baked goods. Honey also works well in sauces, mixed drinks, and marinades that use simple syrup.

- ✔ **Agave nectar:** Use agave nectar, which is lower on the glycemic index than white sugar, in place of sugar and liquid sweeteners. Organic is best because some nonorganic varieties are processed with solvents.

  For recipes that call for white sugar, use two-thirds the amount of agave nectar as you would sugar, and reduce other liquids by ¼ to ⅓ cup. In place of honey or maple syrup, use the same amount of agave. When replacing brown rice syrup, use half to one-third as much agave. And when replacing corn syrup, use half as much agave and increase other liquids by ⅓ cup.

- ✔ **Sorghum, molasses, and brown rice syrup:** You can use these sweeteners in moderation as long as you're not diabetic. Molasses is extracted from the sugar cane. Blackstrap molasses has a distinct flavor and is high in iron, calcium, and potassium — use it as a natural sweetener sparingly with root vegetables, such as squash and pumpkin. Use the same amount of brown rice syrup as you would sugar, but with sorghum and molasses, increase the amount by one-third. For example, if you'd use 1 cup of sugar in a recipe, use 1⅓ cups sorghum or molasses.

Chapter 17

Keeping Your Cool
When Dining Out

*P*eople today are always on the go — shuttling children, going from meeting to meeting, or even going from work to an after-hours get-together. Making meals and dining at home isn't always possible. But dining out — whether you're grabbing fast food or stopping at a sit-down restaurant — doesn't mean your anti-inflammation diet has to go out the window. More restaurants are offering healthier options for entrees, sandwiches, and side dishes in particular.

The key to dining out with inflammation in mind is to pay closer attention to what you're ordering and how it's being prepared. In this chapter, we give you advice on different ways to make wise, healthy choices when eating in a fast-food joint or taking things a little more slowly in a sit-down restaurant.

Choosing a Restaurant

An important first step in dining out is choosing the right door to walk through. It's no secret that the majority of fast food is on the health-food "no" list. Greasy burgers, fried chicken, salty french fries, thick shakes — on their own, each is a nutritional hazard. But put them together, and you've consumed more than a day's worth of trans fats, saturated fats, and sodium, not to mention more calories than you need in one meal. And your body will let you know when enough is enough; too much bad food makes you sluggish and sick, and you'll eventually begin to notice that you're gaining weight.

Even eating out at sit-down restaurants can take a toll on your health — not to mention what it can do to your wallet. Pasta dishes with butter sauce, vegetables cooked in high-fat oils, starches such as potatoes and white rice — there's a plethora of inflammation-inducing hazards just waiting to be set down on your table.

Still, your options for healthy eating can increase greatly if you don't need to go through the drive-through. The menu is broader at sit-down restaurants, for one thing, and the food will be freshly prepared as you order, giving you a better opportunity to control how it's cooked and served.

One thing to keep in mind when selecting a restaurant is knowing which ones use the freshest ingredients, use the most local food, and have the healthiest vegetable choices. Think *locavore* — fresh and local. Foods prepared from fresh ingredients maintain more of their vitamins and health benefits. Try asking around at local markets to identify area restaurants that use local ingredients. Or use websites such as www.organichighways.com, www.organickitchen.com, and www.localharvest.org to help you find locavore restaurants.

Try a vegetarian restaurant or one that serves ethnic foods such as Indian, Thai, or Japanese. These restaurants are typically healthier than most American food restaurants because of the ingredients they use and the number of vegetarian or vegan meal options. The food at these restaurants usually maintains its appearance after it's cooked, which usually means it has kept its nutritional value intact. (For info on ethnic eateries, see the later section "Choosing ethnic fare.")

Regardless of the type of restaurant, make sure your restaurant decisions support your anti-inflammation diet. Know what kinds of foods are available at restaurants and what options you have to avoid inflammation. We discuss menus and food choices in the following sections.

Planning Your Order

When eating out, your job is to make sure you know what you're going to order and why you're ordering it — and then stick with the plan. So what if the others are getting big burgers with the restaurant's special fries on the side? Joining in may make you one of the group, but in terms of suffering inflammatory side effects, you'll be flying solo.

When ordering with a group, try to reach a compromise: They want pizza, but you could do without the added fats from cheeses and most meats, so just choose a veggie pizza to be shared, for example. Or get a salad so you eat less pizza. Want to enjoy the pizza without the guilt? Try a whole-wheat crust or a cheeseless topping, or substitute goat cheese for traditional mozzarella on the top.

TIP

Keeping a healthy social life

Knowing what goes into your meal means you have a better handle on what goes into your body — and just how much of it is anti-inflammatory. That's why the healthiest food in terms of your anti-inflammation diet is the food you make yourself.

But that's not to say eating out is bad, necessarily, as long as you're able to show some restraint and stick to the healthy side of things. After all, the easiest way to slide back into bad habits is to be too restrictive when you're making a change. Depriving yourself of the things that often go along with food, like time with friends, can make things even worse. Letting yourself have a treat, such as a meal out, can give your determination to make the anti-inflammatory diet work a healthy boost.

It's much easier to stick to any change when you can feel like you're not doing it alone, so consider letting yourself go out to lunch with co-workers or out to dinner with friends once a week. Through the remainder of the week, invite people to pack a meal from home and have a picnic when the weather is nice, or get together in the lunch room and have a movie-review discussion. Do you have a full hour for lunch? Bring along a quick board game or a deck of cards and have a short lunch party. That way, you can enjoy better health without missing out on the social benefits of sharing a meal.

When eating at someone else's place for a party, holiday gathering, or potluck, bring an option or two that will fit into your anti-inflammatory diet — but be sure to ask the host whether it's okay to bring something for etiquette's sake. Put together a plate of fresh vegetables with a bean dip or hummus, or bring your own olive oil-based salad dressings with a fresh, seasonal, mixed green salad. For more ideas, check out the recipes in Chapters 9 through 15.

Dining alone? Temptation is still there. To help you stay on track, this section gives you tips on planning your order, whether you're dining solo or in a group.

TIP

Some foods — particularly those higher in fat or that are fried — can make you feel sluggish and bloated, so plan your meal not only for your time at the restaurant but also for the rest of your day. Do you need to stay alert for a meeting or a school event? If so, the healthy options are going to be better all around.

Reading menus and nutritional information

If you're eating out, you want to choose foods that will make both your body and your brain feel good. Knowing which foods are better for you *before* you walk into a restaurant can make your decision-making much easier.

Most restaurants have websites that list their menus; take the time to look up your favorites and see which items fit your new diet. If the website includes nutritional information, know which numbers are important, including how much trans fats, sodium, carbohydrates, protein, and fiber is too much or not enough.

Nutritional claims on menus can be misleading because they're part of food marketing; something may actually be "lower in fat" than it used to be, but that doesn't mean it's healthy. Instead of relying on health statements, take a good look at the menu and find hints for healthy options.

Fried foods in general top the list of *hot* foods that fuel inflammation because of the way they're prepared. Other foods on the hot list include

- Red meats from corn-fed animals
- Partially hydrogenated fats such as those found in margarine and potato chips
- Saturated fats like butter and lard

Many restaurants include how the food is prepared in the description: A grilled chicken breast may be sautéed in oil with onions and garlic, for example, or topped with cheese and sautéed mushrooms. Don't be afraid to ask what kind of oil is used or even whether the chef can skip adding the oil altogether. Try to stay away from vegetable oils and canola oils, and go instead with seed oils such as sunflower and safflower oils.

When looking at the menu, read the item descriptions carefully. Here's what to look for:

- Check for words like *processed* or *cured,* which can mean additives that you don't want. If you're questioning the freshness or even the authenticity of an item (real cheese versus processed cheese, for instance), be sure to ask before ordering.
- *Breaded, batter-dipped,* and *tempura* all mean the same thing: fried. Look instead for baked, poached, boiled, or steamed options. Grilling, broiling, and flame-cooking can cause additional problems, so beware of those preparation methods, as well.
- For sauces, stick to wine or thinned stock-based sauces. Butter sauces, béarnaise, or any sauce that sounds creamy probably is — and is loaded with fat.
- Choose salads with rich, dark greens such as spinach, romaine, or spring mix rather than the pale iceberg. The darker the greens, the more nutrients they have.

One of the most important things to avoid when dealing with inflammation is overcooked foods. Overcooking food of any kind can increase C-reactive protein (CRP) levels and contribute to inflammation. One easy way to avoid this is to ask that meats be cooked no more than "medium" and that vegetables be kept crisp. For example, if you stick your fork into a broccoli spear and lift it off your plate, the spear should still be relatively straight. If it's limp, it's been overcooked.

Considering substitutions and special orders

Just because something is listed as part of a meal on the menu doesn't mean it has to be delivered that way. Consider the meal description as a suggestion rather than an order. That doesn't mean to make a nuisance out of yourself. Rather, look at what's available with other dishes and ask whether you can substitute this for that, or request that the cooks hold the sauces or condiments.

Swapping sides and toppings

Typically speaking, if something is available for one menu item, it's likely available for all of them. Maybe your salmon fillet comes with white rice and steamed vegetables, but the steak your dinner partner is having comes with a potato and a leafy green salad. Ask to substitute a salad for your rice.

When making substitutions, choose vegetables that are prepared in a way that they lose the least amount of nutrients. Broiled or lightly steamed vegetables provide the best levels of much-needed vitamins and nutrients.

Look at your sandwich as well. Does it need to be a sandwich or can you have it without the bun? Are there multi-grain bread options available? Does it come with mayonnaise or another high-fat dressing? Opt instead for extra tomatoes or lettuce. Feel like you need a little something extra on the sandwich? Try a slice of avocado, mustard instead of mayonnaise, or yogurt or cottage cheese instead of sour cream if you can tolerate dairy. You still get that creamy addition but without the fat.

Ordering without the extras

Hold is an important word when keeping a meal healthy — as in "hold the mayo," "hold the gravy," or "hold the sauce." At the very least, if you don't want to skip the sauce entirely, ask to have it on the side, allowing you to control just how much goes onto your meal.

When you're at any kind of restaurant, remember that you're paying for your food and therefore have the right to ask that some of the condiments or other items be removed. Don't be afraid to ask for something the way you want it.

Finding Anti-Inflammatory Foods at Restaurants

Eating out doesn't have to mean eating badly, and you can find healthy options at virtually every kind of restaurant, even fast-food places. The key is to know what foods are inflammatory so that you can avoid them. Ask for substitutions or omissions; for example, ask the kitchen to hold the cheese or the high-fat sauce and ask for something different in its place.

In this section we show you how to make the most of your dining out experience without breaking your new anti-inflammatory lifestyle.

Choosing appetizers and main courses

It's always tempting when looking at a menu to look at the pictures of the appetizers and main courses and make a visual decision about what to order. As with many things, however, giving in to temptation can lead to problems later.

Depending on where you go, most items on the list of appetizers are off-limits unless you can work with the waiter to customize the appetizer. Some restaurants offer an appetizer that blends goat cheese with marinara — but when served with French bread or bruschetta, it takes on a whole new level of fats and sugars.

Being aware of the pitfalls — knowing where the good carbs are, where the dangerous foods may be lurking — can help your anti-inflammatory diet survive a trip to the restaurant. In this section, we give you some suggestions for choosing appetizers and main courses.

Going steamed or baked, not fried

When changing to an anti-inflammatory diet, be sure you know what is good — and what isn't. The wrong kind of fats put many foods in the bad-for-you category, because high fat content can lead to increased cholesterol and triglyceride levels and weight gain and can make foods difficult to digest (see Chapter 5 for details on fats).

The best options for cooking meat in an anti-inflammatory manner are poaching, steaming, and baking; when those options aren't available, grilling and broiling are still better than frying, although cooking at such high temperatures can cause a host of other issues. See Chapter 16 for more information on the hazards of grilling and broiling.

Poaching and steaming meat allow it to retain most of its own natural juices, which keeps the meat from drying out and helps it hold on to its nutritional value. Baking allows the meat to cook slowly rather than a flash-cook like grilling or broiling, again allowing the meat to retain much of its nutritional value.

Frying foods, on the other hand, requires some kind of frying oil, which means added fat. When foods are fried, they absorb a lot of the fat that's in the oils, so even if you're starting off with something healthy, you'll end up with a not-so-healthy item when it's done.

Take a look at the numbers: A salad with fried chicken compared to a salad with baked chicken has 180 more calories (670 versus 490) and 2 extra grams of saturated fat, and that's without the dressing. Side-by-side comparisons of sandwiches are even worse: The fried chicken breast in a sandwich has almost twice the calories and fat as a baked or poached chicken breast in a similar sandwich.

Keeping carbs under control

Carbohydrates often get a bad rap when you're tailoring a diet to meet special needs or even just when creating a healthier menu. But the truth is, you need carbohydrates. Without carbohydrates, your body couldn't make the necessary glucose that gives you energy and really keep it all moving.

The trick is to find good carbohydrates. *Good carbohydrates* usually come in foods with higher fiber and complex carbohydrates — whole grains, nuts and seeds, most vegetables and fruits. The bad carbs usually come from simple carbohydrates (foods with added sugars), foods with high glycemic indexes, or foods that rapidly convert into sugar in the body. Although most fruits and some vegetables have a natural level of sugar, many processed foods have added sugars in the form of high fructose corn syrup or brown sugar.

Drinking for health

Don't think that since you've made all the right food decisions that you're done — you still need to figure out what to drink.

Water is always going to be the best option: There are no additives or calories, and drinking plenty of water during the day is good for hydration, helping you to feel full and "washing out" your insides. Purified, spring, or good tap water are great choices, but mineral waters are best at preventing dehydration because they contain natural electrolytes, such as magnesium, depending on where the water comes from. Add a spritz of lemon or lime to add a little zing.

Want something more than a glass of water? Tea, particularly made from tea leaves rather than a powdered mix combined with something else, provides a healthy dose of antioxidants to your diet to help keep you healthy. In addition, some teas, such as white, green, black, and oolong teas, have been shown to reduce risk of some cancers, including ovarian, skin, and gastric cancers. Green tea can also stimulate *thermogenesis,* which regulates metabolism and may help you lose weight and may lower your blood glucose. Don't be afraid to ask what kind of tea that restaurant serves.

Don't despair, coffee drinkers — moderate consumption of coffee (3 to 5 cups a day) has been shown to reduce your risk of developing Alzheimer's disease and Parkinson's disease and lower the incidence of gallstones and gall bladder attacks.

Stay away from the high-sugar regular sodas, diet sodas made with artificial sweeteners, and other sweetened carbonated beverages. Some restaurants also offer energy drinks or juice drinks, both of which are typically full of sugar and preservatives.

As for alcohol, red wine is a very good choice because of its high levels of antioxidants, but even with wine you'll want to limit consumption. Having a beer or other alcoholic beverage with your meal can be tempting. However, a lot of alcohol is high in sugar and can lead to bad food choices, as can other drinks high in sugar. Artificial sweeteners and sugars trick the mind into craving things you may not really be hungry for, such as fried foods.

Getting your just (and good-for-you) desserts

Just because you're eating healthy doesn't mean you need to avoid the dessert cart. But as with everything else, knowing your limitations can help you make smart choices to help prevent or calm inflammation.

Fruit selections — particularly desserts with fresh fruit — are delicious ways to satisfy your sweet tooth without straying from the healthy lifestyle. A dish of organic, locally grown strawberries and fresh cream is a healthy dessert packed with vitamins and nutrients if you don't have dairy sensitivities. Want to add a little something? Try a plain yogurt parfait with fresh berries and a bit of natural granola.

A fruit sorbet made with fresh fruit, fruit juices, and a natural sweetener can be just what you need for that after-meal treat while providing necessary vitamins to help reduce inflammation and related issues. Want something warm? A baked apple compote with real maple syrup — or without — can be just what you need.

If you're at a restaurant with bakers on staff, the desserts are likely home-made rather than processed. That's good news because it's easier to find out how some of the desserts are made (with butter or shortening, with refined flours and sugars, and so on). Cookies and pie crusts made with butter rather than shortening, especially if it's organic butter, can be fine in moderation — especially in cookies with nuts or in fresh fruit pies.

For many people, ice cream is a year-round favorite. Soft serve is actually less healthy than hard-packed ice cream because of the preservatives used to make it stay soft.

Exploring Food Options by Restaurant Type

You're not always going to know where you'll be eating later, whether it's at a fast-food joint for a quick lunch-on-the-run or a surprise sit-down dinner at your favorite restaurant. Having some prior knowledge about what's available at the various types of restaurants — as well as what you should watch out for — can help you to better enjoy the meal without the unnecessary worry about whether you'll find anything on the menu for you.

Deciding on fast food

Before you get to any fast-food restaurant, do a little homework and find out what each place has to offer. Are their burgers broiled or fried? Does the restaurant offer a salad or fruit as a side alternative? Can you truly "have it your way" in any of them? Most restaurants have nutritional information about their products on their websites or in their restaurants so consumers can make healthier choices.

Here are some tips on choosing fast food:

- ✔ **Burgers:** A regular single-patty burger without mayo or cheese is better than a double anything with the works. Pile on extra vegetables (lettuce and tomato) to take the place of fatty condiments. If given the option, choose a turkey burger instead of a beef burger; turkey is a much leaner meat and scores better on the anti-inflammation checklist. (Even better, opt for a bison burger if it's on the menu.) Choose whole-grain buns over white when possible.

- ✔ **Chicken:** Instead of a breaded and fried chicken sandwich loaded with toppings, order a grilled chicken sandwich with no mayo, for instance, and without the bun. Some fast-food restaurants offer grilled chicken, but inquire about how it's cooked. In many instances, it's still either put into a fryer or fried on a flat grill. Better yet, order baked chicken when it's available.

- ✔ **Subs and sandwiches:** A 6-inch sub is a much better choice than a foot-long sandwich in terms of portion size. Choose lean meats and cheeses with a lot of veggies, and put it all on whole-grain bread. An even better option is to order the sandwich as a whole-grain wrap or as a salad, with all the ingredients on a bed of lettuce.

- ✔ **Burritos and tacos:** It's difficult but not impossible to find anti-inflammatory foods at a fast-food taco or burrito joint. Flour tortillas, corn shells, fried chimichangas, Mexican rice — it all looks like a conspiracy to derail your anti-inflammation plans. But there's hope. Many restaurants offer white-meat chicken as a substitute for the beef in many of their entrees, and some have lean menus, with choices such as chicken tacos with no cheese or sour cream. In some restaurants, you can order a taco or burrito in a bowl without the shell.

- ✔ **Sides:** When possible, choose steamed or stir-fried vegetables — they're full of good carbohydrates because they're packed with fiber, phytochemicals, vitamins, and minerals. Otherwise, go for a side salad or fruit.

A garden salad with grilled chicken and fewer fatty toppings gives you more protein and less fat than one with fried chicken, bacon, and cheese. Keep the dressing low- or nonfat, as well, by using olive oil and vinegar instead of ranch or another creamy dressing.

Choosing ethnic fare

Some ethnic restaurants are better for you than others, with more healthy options on the menu and healthier cooking methods altogether. We've put together a list of recommendations, starting with those with the most options to the fewest:

✔ **East and Southeast Asian:** Asian restaurants have a variety of vegetarian options, and most entrees contain lightly steamed vegetables, something that's at the top of the list of food with anti-inflammatory benefits.

- Japanese choices include miso soup, edamame, and sushi.

- At Chinese restaurants, possibilities are tofu and steamed broccoli or entrees packed with steamed or stir-fried vegetables. Stay away from breaded meats, high-fat dishes like fried rice, and sugary sauces like sweet-and-sour.

- Thai restaurants are great options for vegans and vegetarians with steamed or stir-fried vegetables.

✔ **Indian:** Indian food is a good option for anyone trying to avoid inflammatory foods, as well as for vegans and vegetarians. Entrees with steamed vegetables and brown rice top the list. Although some questions remain about the consumption of ghee, which is clarified butter used in some Indian dishes, it contains no hydrogenated oils. With real ghee, the milk products are removed during the clarifying process, so it's also dairy-free. However, if you have a dairy sensitivity, take care with Indian food to avoid dishes with cream and yogurt.

✔ **Middle Eastern:** Healthy choices include hummus, baba ganoush, grilled chicken, and entrees with steamed vegetables and whole-grain rice.

✔ **Mediterranean:** Even though Mediterranean food tops the list for foods with anti-inflammatory benefits, finding restaurants that include the best of anti-inflammatory options is often hard. At Greek restaurants, look for Greek salad, bean dishes, fish, and vegetables.

✔ **Italian:** Go for the bean dishes and those with fish and vegetables. Avoid the bread, and skip menu items that are *frito,* or fried, and instead choose *griglia,* or grilled, dishes. Avoid Alfredo dishes, which come with a heavy cream and butter-based sauce loaded with fat and calories; marinara dishes are typically tomato- and vegetable-based and are considerably lower in both fat and calories.

✔ **Mexican:** The best anti-inflammatory options on the menu are guacamole and dishes with real beans — not refried — and fish. Avoid fried foods.

Keeping Portions Under Control

Restaurants keep increasing the size of their portions — look at how many have mega-size pizzas or supersized meals. Ever look at a plate of food that's just arrived and thought, "I'll never be able to eat all of that"? If it looks like too much food, it probably is.

Sometimes your mother was wrong — you don't have to clean your plate. Instead of tempting your taste buds into finishing it all, ask the server right away for a take-home box and put half your meal away before you take that first bite. Don't like taking food home? Offer to split a meal with a friend.

Don't confuse portions with servings. A *portion* is the amount of food that's on your plate, and a *serving* is the right amount of food to eat at a sitting. You're the only one in control of the size of your serving — don't rely on the restaurant to do it for you. Here are some serving-size guidelines to keep in mind when considering portions:

- One serving of whole-grain bread is equal to one slice. If you're having a full sandwich, that's two servings.

- A serving of cooked vegetables is about ½ cup. You're not likely to bring a measuring cup to dinner, but keep in mind that one serving of fruits or vegetables is about the size of your fist.

- A serving of pasta is about the size of a scoop of ice cream. Think about the last time you went to an Italian restaurant — how much pasta was on your plate?

- A serving of fish or chicken is 3 ounces and is about the size of a deck of cards.

Chapter 18

Looking at Prescription-Drug Alternatives and Supplements

*I*n addition to refining your diet, finding supplements to boost your immune system and keep inflammation at bay can keep you feeling your best. Over-the-counter drugs may also offer temporary relief.

Pharmaceutical *drugs,* which are generally synthetic creations of laboratory work, are designed to prevent or treat a particular condition. Drugs are generally developed to be potent and to work *for* the body; they therefore have not only strong activity but also some potentially strong side effects. Herbs and supplements, on the other hand, generally work *with* the body because they contain dietary ingredients — compounds that are recognized by the body based on the food you eat (vitamins, minerals, phytochemicals, and so on).

That's not to say that there's always a clear line between drugs and supplements. Herbal medicine is the oldest system of medicine. In fact, many drugs were initially derived from plants and were later synthesized in the lab for consistency of the *active constituents* (chemical compounds that do what the drug is supposed to be used for).

In this chapter, we talk about over-the-counter drugs (particularly anti-inflammatory drugs such as NSAIDs), discuss some supplements you may want to consider, and give you some guidelines on choosing supplements wisely.

Treating Inflammation with Over-the-Counter Medication

Americans have become a society of pill-poppers. Take a walk through the drugstore or the health section of any grocery store, and you see a medication for almost every ailment imaginable. If there's no specific pill, there's always the multi-use acetaminophen or ibuprophen or naproxen to take for everything from a headache to a pulled muscle. Aspirin therapy — in which patients take an aspirin dose every day — is a popular regimen for people who have or who want to avoid heart disease.

Drugs tend to be powerful and fast-acting, so pharmaceutical medications that relieve pain or decrease inflammation may be helpful short-term. However, medication can have long-term consequences. Over-the-counter medications like acetaminophen (Tylenol) caution users with liver damage not to take the drug because it may make the situation worse. Children who show signs of chicken pox or the flu and take aspirin face a substantial risk of developing *Reye's syndrome*, which can cause acute brain damage and create problems with liver function. Get to prescription medication, which is stronger, and some of the side effects worsen.

Still, anti-inflammatory drugs can be very useful — or even necessary when prescribed by your medical doctor — when diet alone isn't the answer. In this section, we discuss some over-the-counter pain-relievers and anti-inflammatory drugs, and we cover aspirin therapy in people with heart disease.

Medication should not replace lifestyle changes in diet and exercise. An anti-inflammatory diet can complement the activity of a drug and may even help you to use less of or get off the medication. Make sure your physician follows your progress, and never stop a medication without consulting with your physician.

Exploring how anti-inflammatory drugs work

Inflammation doesn't just happen. Your body's cells send out signals to cell receptors, and how those receptors interpret what they're being told may lead to inflammation. For example, your body produces *prostaglandins*, chemicals that promote inflammation, soreness, and fever to get the immune system's defenses going to fight infection or illness.

Prostaglandins are produced by the *cyclooxygenase* (COX) enzyme, and there are two such enzymes: COX-1 and COX-2. Drugs that work to block or reduce inflammation — nonsteroidal anti-inflammatory drugs (NSAIDs) — do so by blocking the COX enzymes and reducing the prostaglandins.

The COX-1 enzyme also produces prostaglandins that support platelets and protect the stomach. Using NSAIDs also reduces these prostaglandins, which can cause ulcers and other issues.

Navigating your way through over-the-counter drugs

One type of pain reliever is acetaminophen, commonly sold as Tylenol or Panadol. In some cases, acetaminophen pain relievers also contain caffeine or decongestants and are promoted to treat a combination of symptoms, most often as cold relief or flu relief, and may treat a runny nose or chest congestion in addition to the pain. Acetaminophen relieves pain and reduces fevers but doesn't fight inflammation.

Most over-the-counter pain relievers are NSAIDs — *nonsteroidal anti-inflammatory drugs*. NSAIDs relieve the pain and reduce swelling of inflammation. Generally speaking, ibuprofen, naproxen, and ketoprofen (sold as Advil, Aleve, and Orudis, respectively) do a better job of relieving pain than acetaminophen or aspirin, but the other drugs have their own advantages. Doctors often suggest acetaminophen for arthritis relief because it's gentler on the stomach, and aspirin does have some effect on the risks of heart attack (see the next section for details).

There are several different categories of NSAIDs, including salicylic acids, propionic acids, acetic acids, enolic acids, fenamic acids, napthylalkanones, pyranocarboxylic acids, pyrroles, and COX-2 inhibitors. Talk to your doctor or physician to get an idea of which one may be right for you.

Although a variety of prescription and nonprescription anti-inflammatory medications are available, there's no real proof that one is better or stronger than any other. Differences lie instead in how individual inflammation sufferers respond to various medications and the risks for side effects. Some people may be able to take the NSAIDs like ibuprofen or naproxen without incident, and others may need something milder and that doesn't upset their digestive systems or cause other problems.

Using aspirin for heart disease: Take two and call me in the morning

Almost everyone's heard of the benefits of aspirin in heart patients. For people who've had cardiovascular events — a heart attack, for example — taking an aspirin a day helps reduce the risk of a recurrence.

Aspirin works by interfering in your blood's clotting capabilities. With *atherosclerosis*, your arteries begin to narrow because of a buildup of fatty deposits, commonly referred to as hardening of the arteries, and those fatty deposits can burst. A blood clot then forms and can block the artery or can detach and move elsewhere in the circulatory system, preventing blood flow to the heart or the brain and causing a heart attack or stroke. Aspirin acts as a blood thinner, keeping the blood from clotting and possibly preventing the blockage of the artery.

According to the Mayo Clinic, aspirin therapy has different effects on men and women. In men of all ages, an aspirin a day may prevent a first and second heart attack and reduce the risk of heart disease. In women under age 65, taking an aspirin daily can prevent a first stroke and a second heart attack and help reduce the risk of heart disease. In women over age 65, aspirin therapy can do all that as well as prevent a first heart attack. That's the good news about aspirin therapy.

Daily aspirin therapy isn't for everyone. If you've never had a heart attack or stroke, taking a preventative daily aspirin could actually create a larger danger than the heart attack or stroke. In 2009, about 50 million Americans were taking low-dose aspirin — 325 milligrams or less — a day to prevent heart disease. Some had had prior cardiovascular events or stroke, but many were taking the pills as a *primary preventive* measure. Researchers discovered, however, that daily use of aspirin for those who hadn't had a heart attack or stroke was not only unnecessary but posed certain health risks of its own, including the potential for causing a hemorrhagic stroke (which is a rupture of a blood vessel in the brain) or intestinal bleeding.

Before stopping daily aspirin therapy, discuss your options with your physician. A sudden stop in medication can trigger a heart attack or stroke.

You can use omega-3 fatty acids, found in fish or fish oil, to do some of the same things as aspirin but without all the unwanted side effects. Omega-3 fatty acids reduce pain, prevent platelet aggregation, and lower the risk of heart attacks and stroke.

Using Dietary Supplements to Fill in the Nutritional Gaps

According to the Food and Drug Administration (FDA), a *dietary supplement* is "a product taken by mouth that contains a 'dietary ingredient' intended to supplement the diet." A supplement may include anything that's naturally derived that is not a drug, including vitamins, minerals, herbs, amino acids, and some naturally derived hormone-like substances.

Supplements generally aren't as fast-acting as drugs, but some supplements are just as effective without the side effects. Supplements tend to be safer for long-term use. Vitamins and minerals such as calcium, magnesium, and vitamin D are used on a daily basis. People may use herbs and supplements short-term for acute issues (echinacea for colds), as a substitute for pharmaceutical medication (red yeast rice for statins, which lower cholesterol), and short-term or long-term for medical conditions (quercetin for acute allergies).

This section covers some supplements you may want to consider.

Not all supplements are safe, and you can face problems if you don't know how to take supplements correctly. Work with a physician or herbalist who's been trained in drug, nutrient, and food interactions. We discuss choosing supplements safely later in "Choosing Dietary Supplements Wisely."

Taking vitamins as a defense against inflammation

We're sure you've heard it: Don't forget to take your vitamins! By increasing your daily intake of vitamins — either through supplements or by eating more of the foods that contain them — you can help keep inflammation at bay and curb the pain of existing inflammation.

Getting all the vitamins you need from food can be difficult, so consider taking a multivitamin (ask your doctor about the right kind and amount for you). Multivitamins have been shown to decrease the risk of hospitalizations and many diseases, thereby helping to reduce healthcare costs.

A vitamin's recommended daily dosage means the amount of the vitamin needed to prevent a deficiency, but that amount doesn't give you therapeutic nor optimal benefits. Always consult with your physician before taking high doses of vitamins and minerals because they can cause other nutrient imbalances or be potentially toxic.

B vitamins

B vitamins, particularly B6, B9 (folic acid), and B12, are high on the list of vitamins that have heart-protective properties. B6 is also prescribed to arthritis sufferers because at high doses, it shrinks the inflamed membranes around the arthritis-affected joints.

Food sources of B vitamins vary according to each vitamin: B1, also called thiamin, is in egg yolks, whole-grain breads, brown rice, green leafy vegetables, and legumes; B2, or riboflavin, is in eggs, milk, whole-grain products, and peas; B3, or niacin, is in meats, eggs, legumes, peanuts, fish, and potatoes; B6, or pyridoxine, is in liver, meat, brown rice, fish, butter, wheat germ, and soybeans; B9, or folic acid, is in green vegetables, liver, and whole-grain cereals; and B12 is in liver, meat, egg yolk, poultry, and milk.

Vitamin D

Vitamin D helps slow or prevent osteoporosis, high blood pressure, cancer, and several autoimmune diseases. It aids in the absorption of calcium, which helps the body maintain strong, healthy bones. The benefits of vitamin D also show up in the dentist's chair, reducing gingivitis (inflammation of the gums).

The best source of vitamin D is unfiltered sunlight, which triggers your skin to make its own vitamin D. Good dietary sources of vitamin D include coldwater oily fish such as sardines, herring, and wild salmon.

Vitamin E

Vitamin E has powerful anti-inflammatory properties. It's been clinically proven to help reduce the risk of heart disease, Alzheimer's, arthritis, and hay fever.

The recommended daily dosage of vitamin E is about 30 International Units (IU), or about 20 milligrams. A general daily dose of 400 IU mixed tocopherols may be helpful in reducing oxidation.

Alpha-tocopherol, one of the forms of vitamin E, and synthetic forms of vitamin E actually increase risk of heart disease when you take them in high amounts. Be sure to look for "mixed tocopherols" and nonsynthetic vitamin E. Mixed tocopherols are a mixture of the natural forms of vitamin E found in food, such as almonds.

Too much vitamin E has been linked to increased instances of bleeding. Although everyone should check with his or her medical practitioner before starting any kind of supplement or vitamin program, people who take blood-thinning medication or who have vitamin K deficiency should take particular caution.

Finding the benefits of fish oil tablets

Fish oil can be a healthy lifestyle addition. Fish oil is filled with the essential omega-3 fatty acids and provides health benefits for a variety of issues, from heart disease and cancer to eye disorders and skin care. Here are a few of the areas omega-3s affect:

- ✔ **Brain function:** The presence of omega-3 fatty acids in fish oils has a mood stabilizing effect, calming anxiety and depression and treating bipolar disorder. These good fats are especially important in helping the brain's cells, or *neurons,* to signal each other effectively, so omega-3s also help control Alzheimer's disease. DHA also plays a role in serotonin and dopamine metabolism, having a positive effect on mood.

- ✔ **Obesity and heart health:** Omega-3s can help alleviate the problems associated with obesity, including heart disease and diabetes. The American Heart Association touts fish oil as playing a vital role in reducing the risk of heart disease by lowering the LDL (bad) cholesterol and raising the HDL (good) cholesterol and preventing triglycerides from getting out of control. Fish oils prevent platelet aggregation (they act as blood thinners) and help with heart arrhythmias.

- ✔ **Gastrointestinal disorders:** Fish oil is anti-inflammatory and has proven effective in the treatment and prevention of gastrointestinal disorders like Crohn's disease, ulcerative colitis, and irritable bowel disorders (IBD).

- ✔ **Immune system:** Research suggests that making fish oil a regular part of your diet can boost your immune system, and help reduce the risk of inflammation in rheumatoid arthritis and autoimmune diseases.

The best natural sources of fish oil are, not surprisingly, fish. The problem with fresh fish, however, is that thanks to pollutants such as mercury, arsenic, lead, PCBs (polychlorinated biphenyls), and other substances in the waters, the oils found in fish are often contaminated.

Pharmaceutical grade fish oils are a supplement that most physicians, holistic or otherwise, can agree on as being an important supplement for reducing the risk of cardiovascular disease and inflammation. Fish oil tablets, particularly those of good quality, provide a more than adequate substitute for the real thing, allowing your body to get the full benefits of the essential omega-3 fatty acids. To get a good quality fish oil, choose a brand that's tested for heavy metals, that's shelf stable, and that isn't synthetic (see Chapter 22).

Fish oils do not have the toxic side effects on the gastrointestinal system and liver that the pharmaceutical drugs like aspirin do because they have more of a generalized anti-inflammatory benefit rather than targeting a specific pathway; targeting a specific pathway increases the potential for side effects.

Getting a boost from mighty magnesium

You'd be hard-pressed to find a system in your body that doesn't depend on magnesium. It plays important roles in the health of your cardiovascular, digestive, muscular, skeletal, and nervous systems, as well as your brain, kidneys, and liver. Magnesium helps blood pressure stay low, serves as a bone strengthener, and can help alleviate problems associated with metabolic disorder — obesity, diabetes, and high cholesterol levels. More than 300 enzymes in the body need magnesium to ensure they're doing their jobs properly.

Studies show that a deficiency in magnesium can lead to elevated C-reactive protein (CRP) levels, which can in turn lead to heart disease and other inflammatory diseases (see Chapter 3 for details). That said, the majority of Americans — a whopping 68 percent — don't even come close to getting the recommended daily allowance (RDA) of magnesium. Some of the signs of magnesium deficiency are muscle weakness, heart arrhythmia, headaches, elevated blood pressure, depression, nausea, vomiting, and lack of appetite.

Some of the best dietary sources for magnesium are spinach, Swiss chard, mustard greens, broccoli, and summer squash. It's also available in a supplement form, both in *chelated* and *nonchelated* (connected with another molecule or not connected) forms. There are many forms of magnesium, but magnesium citrate is well absorbed and doesn't create loose stools as may occur with other forms.

An overabundance of magnesium can lead to magnesium toxicity, symptoms of which include diarrhea, drowsiness, and weakness. Be sure to check with a healthcare provider before starting on any supplemental form. The safest way to get a boost in magnesium is through your diet.

Taking herbal supplements and spices

Many herbs and spices don't just add a little zing to the flavor of your food; they also provide a flurry of anti-inflammatory benefits, from putting an end to migraines to reducing your risk of certain cancers and heart disease. Knowing what to use and how to use herbs and spices is one big step in the fight against inflammation (see Chapter 22 for details on the ten most powerful natural supplements).

Most herbs and spices are available in food form, as well as in capsules and tincture. Food form is the safest and easiest to find.

Here's a list of some of the most common herbs and spices with anti-inflammatory benefits:

✔ **Ginger:** Ginger calms an ailing stomach and is a safe end to vomiting during pregnancy, but its healthful benefits go much further. Ginger contains very powerful anti-inflammatory compounds called *gingerols* that help relieve the pain of arthritis and osteoarthritis. Those same gingerols provide a protection against colorectal cancer and ovarian cancer. (We discuss ginger more in Chapter 22.)

✔ **Turmeric:** This spice was first used as a dye in India more than 2,500 years ago, but it's now a common ingredient in many Indian dishes. Turmeric is one of the most powerful natural spices available, with anti-cancer properties that work against pancreatic, colon and breast cancer as well as melanoma and leukemia. Turmeric helps fight Alzheimer's disease and multiple sclerosis, and it works as a natural painkiller and antibacterial agent when used as a disinfectant for cuts and burns. (You can find more information about turmeric in Chapter 22.)

✔ **Aloe vera:** Aloe vera has long been known for its soothing properties in healing external cuts and sunburns, but it has some pretty powerful anti-inflammatory benefits when ingested, as well. Aloe vera can cool inflammation in the digestive tract, as with peptic ulcers, and has been used to quell problems with the liver in some countries, such as China. Take caution, however: Aloe vera can cause hypoglycemia and have a laxative effect. It counteracts with some medications, so consult with a health care provider before taking aloe vera.

✔ **Licorice:** Licorice has healing qualities for colds and coughs, and it also works against chronic hepatitis. People with elevated blood pressure should take caution, however; too much licorice may increase blood pressure in some people when used long term. For this reason, holistic practitioners frequently use a form of licorice root that's had *glycyrrhizin,* the part that may increase blood pressure, removed.

✔ **Boswellia:** Boswellia helps provide joint support and helps prevent arthritis. Some people suggest it as an herbal remedy for Crohn's disease, asthma, and colitis. (Turn to Chapter 22 for more coverage of the benefits of boswellia.)

Choosing Dietary Supplements Wisely

More and more people are turning to nutritional supplements to either battle inflammatory issues they're at risk for or just give themselves a bit of a healthy boost. You can see evidence of the growing number of people looking for supplements on the store shelves: the number of companies producing supplements seems to grow every day.

But like pharmaceutical drugs, supplements present dangers of unsafe inter-actions or incorrect dosages. Despite all their healthy anti-inflammatory benefits, if you take too much of any supplement, you stand a good chance of doing more harm than good.

Trying to self-prescribe supplements and deciding on your own dosage is dangerous. Always turn to a healthcare provider before starting any kind of supplement to make sure it's the right one for you and that it won't react with other medications, your diet, or anything else in your lifestyle.

In this section, we outline how an expert can help you decide which supple-ments to choose and how much to take. We also show you how to read labels correctly so you know that what you're picking up is what you really want.

Getting some professional guidance

Consult a naturopathic physician or other medical expert who's specifically trained in nutrition and dietary and herbal supplements. Here are some things your Naturopath or other dietary expert can help with:

- ✓ **Which supplements are safe and effective:** Drugs are closely regulated by the Food and Drug Administration (FDA) and must go through rigor-ous and expensive laboratory and clinical trials before they can be put on the market. However, because herbs and supplements do not require FDA approval, you rarely see much clinical research on their activity or benefits. An expert can tell you which supplements likely do what they're supposed to.

- ✓ **Specific type of supplement:** Maybe you read in a magazine that echi-nacea is good for colds, but did you know there are many species of echinacea and that not all of them work effectively as an immune system booster? A naturopathic physician has had at least four years' training in herbal medicine as part of his or her medical school education.

- ✓ **Ingredients:** You don't know what you're getting when you pick up supplements from someone other than a professional, and you can do more harm than good by taking a product over-the-counter. Fish oils, for example, are good for your heart and may help lower cholesterol, but taking a poor quality fish oil may actually increase your cholesterol by causing further oxidation rather than preventing oxidation.

    Your physician can guide you toward quality products. Sometimes qual-ity means paying more for what you need, but the real question is this: Do you want to pay for your health now or later? If you penny-pinch on supplements, you may be setting yourself up to spend much more in hospital bills later.

✔ **Possible interactions and side effects:** Herbs and supplements, although generally safer than pharmaceutical drugs, do have potential side effects and can interact with other supplements and medications. An expert can tell you which supplements interact with medication and can help you through any problems.

✔ **Proper dosage:** More isn't necessarily better. Ingesting too much of a certain vitamin or supplement can be dangerous. For example, some supplements may boast 500 percent of the recommended daily value of vitamin C, but too much vitamin C can cause diarrhea and dehydration, and an overabundance of some B vitamins can cause temporary nerve damage, including tingling in the hands and feet. Be sure to consider how much of each nutrient you're getting through your diet when determining the dosage of a supplement. Turn to your Naturopath or other medical professional to find out how much to take.

✔ **Individualized treatment:** Your physician can help make sure you get the right combination for your genetics, biochemical individuality, and lifestyle. Just as your fingerprints are unique, so is the way your body works. Have a professional assess your case for an optimal treatment plan.

Not all states or Canadian provinces have licensure for naturopathic doctors, so some individuals use the title without the four-year medical education. Seek out a practitioner who got his or her degree from an accredited school and not an online program. Two websites that can help you find a licensed naturopathic doctor are www.naturopathic.org and www.cand.ca.

Understanding labels

After you consult with a physician (making sure you ask which retailers have the best quality supplements), pick up the bottle, look at the label, and ask these two key questions:

✔ **Where do the nutrients come from?** Like other food products, dietary supplements have a nutritional label with the ingredients listed. Some manufacturers put the source of the nutrient next to the ingredient. Recognize any of the names? You should be able to recognize and pronounce most if not all of the ingredients and sources.

✔ **Does it have natural or artificial ingredients?** Just as you don't want to eat artificial sugars or refined flours, you want your supplements to be natural with no artificial or chemical ingredients. Even if the ingredient is a derivative of the whole product, you're losing some of the value of the whole nutrient. For example, are there artificial colors or additives like sodium lauryl sulfate or propylene glycol? These ingredients have no health benefits; they just make the product appear more appealing.

Considering quality standards

Not all supplements are created equal. Although pharmaceutical drugs have standardized formulas, supplements can vary in their composition. With whole plant extracts, for example, the amount of the *active constituent* (effective ingredient) that the plant produces will vary; some companies created standardized extracts for this reason. There's controversy in the herbal medicine industry because sometimes the stated amount of the active compound is inaccurate, such as with hypericin in St. John's wort. Similarly, two bottles both saying they contain ginger may have varying levels of actual ginger, supplemented themselves with chemicals or other additives in an effort to make the product — though not necessarily the ginger — last longer.

There are no strict standards on quality of ingredients for nutritional supplements and herbs, so many products lack clinical effectiveness. The FDA (www.fda.gov) is trying to improve standards with their updated Dietary Supplements Health and Education Act (DSHEA) through improving good manufacturing practices (GMP). However, there's no substitute for expert advice.

When searching for the best quality supplements, take these first steps:

- ✔ **Do your research.** Go online and check reputable sources — the Better Business Bureau, the Food and Drug Administration, and the U.S. Department of Agriculture, for starters — to see what they may say about various herbs and supplements. Then check company websites — see what they say about their research and quality standards. Are they promoting the quality of the product or the fact that it's the cheapest on the market? Have their products been tested by an independent lab?

    If something sounds too good to be true, it probably is. If a supplement guarantees it will make you lose X number of pounds in 30 days, be wary. Every person's body responds to each supplement in its own way; there's no real way to know for how long — or whether — a supplement will work for you. Be wary of anecdotal "testimonials" about amazing results or of anything that claims to be "totally safe."

- ✔ **Look for the expiration date.** This sounds like a simple step, but you'd be surprised by the number of people who don't realize supplements expire. Don't take expired supplements expecting to get the full nutritional value. Things that contain oils may go rancid beyond their effectiveness date, particularly if they've been exposed to heat and/or light.

✔ **Check with the store.** Avoid going to price clubs or pharmacies for nutritional supplements; you can generally find better-quality supplements in your physician's office or at a health food store. Your health-care provider should be recommending a specific brand. See what the health food store's on-duty nutritionist or other expert knows about a certain company or brand. If a product is good quality, the staff will likely know about it. The quality of the product is generally reflected in the price.

Don't shop online for vitamins, herbs, or supplements. You don't know what you're getting, and a lot of scams are out there. Even though the label looks good, there's no guarantee the bottle will have anything useful in it.

Chapter 19

Making Strides Against Inflammation

In This Chapter

▶ Working with cardiovascular workouts

▶ Looking at the basics of meditation and yoga

You've taken steps to get inflammatory foods out of your life. Now you're ready to turn not only to an anti-inflammatory diet but to an anti-inflammatory *lifestyle*. To do that, you need to look at ways to get your heart pumping and keep your body moving. Keeping your body moving through exercise is an important part of the healing and regenerative process, and skipping exercise is a sure way to allow inflammation to stick around and significantly delay the healing process. Calming exercises such as yoga further reduce inflammation by reducing stress.

The gentle aerobic exercises, meditations, and yoga moves in this chapter can help jump-start your body in its physical fight against inflammation.

Fighting Inflammation with Cardiovascular Activity

Sticking to a regular high-intensity workout that's short in duration — about 15 to 30 minutes — reduces your risks of obesity and therefore your risks of metabolic syndrome (see Chapter 3 for the links between inflammation and chronic disease). Physical exercise is also associated with decreased risk of cardiovascular and heart disease. Exercise promotes the release of feel-good endorphins, helps the immune system (when you don't overdo it), helps with weight loss and maintenance, and is a great stress reliever. Increased blood flow and sweating enhance detoxification, and exercise helps your body use sugars instead of storing them in the liver, which helps improve problems with insulin resistance.

Furthermore, building and maintaining lean muscle mass helps your metabolism to function optimally and helps reduce inflammation. Lean muscle mass, rather than fat, helps with inflammation because excess fat cells cause toxicity and inflammatory disruption in the signals of the endocrine system.

In this section, we introduce ways you can get the blood flowing and build a little muscle in the process.

 Remember to stretch before and after every workout. Stretching has a way of fooling your muscles into thinking they're already or still working, enhancing the benefits of your workout by up to 20 percent. Stretching also helps your muscles begin to contract more smoothly, alleviating some of the pain you may feel early on.

Starting off simply with walking and swimming

Walking is the best place to start, particularly because it's something you likely do to some degree every day. Walking is an easy and excellent way to boost your heart rate, it's easier on your joints than running, and it's something you can do at any time. Walk around the house in inclement weather, or go up and down the stairs a few times. Better yet, get a treadmill and walk for miles, even when it's raining.

 The best way to make an exercise routine stick is to find a way to make it enjoyable. When you're walking, find a pleasant route with great things to see or one that makes you feel comfortable and relaxed. With other exercises, try playing some upbeat music or exercising with friends.

 Integrate more walking into your routine by doing so gradually. Keep a pedometer handy and work weekly to boost the number of steps you take each day. If you're walking 2,000 steps now, for example, shoot for 2,500 next week. Keep that up for a week and then shoot for another 500-step boost.

Swimming is another great way to get your heart pumping. The water works to soothe the joints rather than put extra stress on them, so swimming is therapeutic as well as aerobic. If you have access to a pool, try to incorporate 30 minutes of swimming into your routine three to four times a week.

When you get your body ready, you can step the workout up a notch, being sure to incorporate 30 minutes of exercise into your day at least three times a week.

Get it going good: Stimulating exercises

The following sections guide you through a few moves that are sure to get your heart going. Be sure to have an exercise mat and plenty of room to get the most out of your workout. Doing these exercises in sequence is a great start to a good fitness routine, and altogether you'll have about a 20-minute workout. Don't be afraid to do each exercise a little longer or find another to add to the routine if you want to stretch your workout to 30 minutes.

Squat thrusts

These squat thrusts are a great way to start your exercise routine and get your heart rate nice and high while working your entire body.

1. **Stand with your feet about hip-width apart.**
2. **Squat to the floor, placing your hands directly in front of you and about shoulder-width apart.**
3. **With your weight on your arms, very quickly jump your feet behind you so that you're in a push-up position; then jump back and stand up.**

Try to do 10 repetitions within a minute. Pause for 30 seconds and then do another set of 10. Pause for another 30 seconds and do a third set of 10.

If your inflammation is in your knees or hips, be sure to consult a physician before trying squat thrusts, and start with shorter, slower repetitions.

Mountain climbers

As with squat thrusts, mountain climbers raise your heart rate rather quickly.

1. **Begin in a push-up position with your legs out straight.**
2. **Bring your right knee in to your chest, resting your foot on the floor.**
3. **Quickly jump and switch legs, returning the right leg to a straight line and bringing the left knee up.**

Continue alternating legs as quickly as you can for a full minute. Pause for 30 seconds and repeat for another minute. Take another 30-second break before doing a final minute of mountain climbers.

Be sure to consult a physician if your inflammation is in your legs, because mountain climbers may exacerbate rather than relieve some of the pain.

Deep squat lunges

These lunges are great for raising your heart rate without the added pressure on your knees and hips. If you have inflammation in your legs, these lunges will aid in the healing process without risking re-injury.

1. **Stand with your feet shoulder-width apart, arms at your sides.**

2. **Step your left foot out to the left, bending your left knee and extending your right leg in a side lunge.**

   As you lunge to the left, raise your right arm over your head and reach left. Bring your left arm across your hips and reach right, as shown in Figure 19-1a. Be careful not to let your left knee extend past your toes.

3. **Return to your starting position, with feet shoulder-width apart and arms at your sides.**

4. **Repeat Step 2, this time lunging to the right and reaching your left arm up and over your head, as shown in Figure 19-1b.**

5. **Return to your starting position.**

6. **Continue lunges for 5 minutes, alternating sides.**

   Try to stretch a little farther with each lunge.

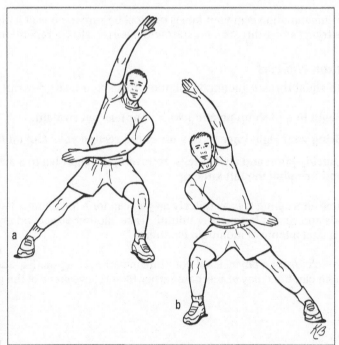

Figure 19-1: Lunge to the left, and then to the right.

Invisible jump rope

This exercise raises your heart rate and lets you control how quickly it climbs based on how fast you jump.

1. **Stand upright with your feet hip-width apart. Keeping elbows at your sides, pretend you're holding a jump rope.**

2. **Begin twirling "the rope" and jumping.**

3. **Continue for five minutes, varying speeds.**

Be careful if you're having trouble with your knees, because the bouncing can create a painful impact.

Slowing it down: Relaxing moves

Not quite ready for moving fast, or need something to help you cool down? Here are a few moves that keep your heart rate up without putting strain on your joints.

Intermittent leg lifts

These leg lifts are a much less aerobic move than some exercises and therefore shouldn't cause additional strain on any of your joints. It's a great starter move for people who suffer inflammation pain in the hips and/or knees.

1. **Lie on your back on your exercise mat, arms at your sides with hands flat.**

2. **Keeping your legs together, raise your feet 6 inches; hold them up for 10 seconds.**

3. **Pressing your hands to the floor for support, raise your feet another 6 inches and hold for 10 seconds.**

4. **Again pressing your hands to the floor for support, raise your feet one more time, this time so your legs and torso form a right angle; hold for 10 seconds.**

5. **Slowly begin lowering your feet, holding your feet 12 inches off the ground for 10 seconds and at 6 inches for 10 seconds.**

6. **When your feet are back on the floor, rest for 15 seconds and repeat.**

   Perform this exercise four times.

After you get this move mastered, add some variation by holding a ball between your feet as you raise your legs. First use a playground ball, and then up in size until eventually you work with a stabilizer ball.

Stabilizing ab crunch

This ab crunch is a great exercise to help reduce some of that dangerous belly fat while at the same time increasing your heart rate. The stability ball provides support to your lower back.

1. Get out your stability ball and put it on the center of your exercise mat.

2. Stand in front of the ball with your feet at shoulder-width apart.

3. Lower yourself so that you're sitting on the ball.

4. Cross your arms over your chest or clasp your hands gently behind your head and lie back, letting your back curve slightly with the ball.

5. Slowly rise so that your shoulders come up off the ball, as shown in Figure 19-2.

6. Repeat. Do 10 crunches, slowing increasing by 5 crunches over time.

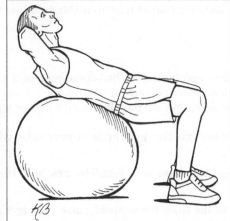

Figure 19-2:
The stability ball supports your back as you crunch.

Finding Stress Relief in Meditation and Yoga

Everyone experiences a little bit of stress, and when you're facing health issues or making big changes, that stress level can slowly inch upward until you feel tense, jittery, and just plain uncomfortable. Stress is a cause of inflammation; when too much of it occurs for too long, your body's natural anti-inflammatory hormone, cortisol, gets out of balance.

For generations, people have used meditation and yoga to help the body naturally relieve stress and become centered and relaxed.

Centering yourself through meditation

Avoiding all stress is impossible, but knowing how to deal with stress helps make the knot seem much smaller. For years relaxation experts have turned to *centering,* a form of meditation that involves deep breathing, slowing down your heart rate, and relaxing your muscles. Meditation can help lower blood pressure and relieve insomnia and anxiety by reducing adrenaline levels and increasing the amount of serotonin released into the body. *Serotonin,* the "happy hormone," plays a key role in determining mood and anxiety levels — the more serotonin, the better the mood and the lower the anxiety.

Not only does meditation allow you to take a break from your day to quiet your mind and body, but research also shows that meditation prevents premature aging of the brain — the effects of aging on things like memory, cognitive function, and responses.

Setting up and breathing

The first step in preparing for an optimum meditation is to ensure you have a clean, quiet space. Meditation is a way of decluttering your mind, so make sure the space around you isn't filled with clutter, either.

Lay your exercise mat out flat. Light a scented candle or some incense, or use a few drops of essential oil in a diffuser to help turn down the stress, and your inflammation along with it. Lavender helps with sleep and relaxation, and sandalwood can help with meditation.

Sit with your back straight and your feet flat on the floor. Close your eyes and take three deep, slow breaths. Focus your mind on your feet; imagine them slowly sending roots into the ground. As you exhale, envision yourself sending all your negative energy down through the roots into the earth. With each inhale, imagine bringing positive energy up from the ground into your body. Picture the positive energy coming to you in the form of a white light, cresting on your crown.

Continue this breathing exercise until you feel your stress levels lowering.

Chakra

The chakra meditation is a breathing exercise in which you focus on a different *chakra,* or part of your body, with each cleansing breath. The *chakra* — the Hindu word for "wheel" or "turning" — is the concept of *force centers,* spinning receptors of energy permeating the layers of the body.

Different systems have a varying number of chakras, but the most popular in the Western world is the system of seven chakras (you start with the first):

1. Base of the spine

2. Sexual organs

3. Stomach

4. Heart

5. Throat

6. "Third eye" (brow)

7. Head

When doing a chakra meditation, begin by laying your yoga mat out flat and lighting a scented candle or some incense. Lavender helps with sleep and relaxation, and sandalwood can help with meditation. Sit or lie down with your back straight and your feet flat on the floor. Close your eyes and take three deep, slow breaths.

After you've relaxed, imagine a colorful ball of energy pushing up through the earth and to your spine (the first chakra). The color of the light is up to you, but it should be a color that you feel represents your energy.

As you breathe, imagine the ball of energy hovering over each of your chakras, cleansing the area of negative energy and boosting it with positive energy and relaxation. With each stop, the ball pushes the negativity up toward the sky.

When you reach the seventh chakra, the head, let go of your ball of light and feel positive energy — a feel-good factor — pushing up through you, again through the chakra process. Positive energy comes from concentrating on positive things and pushing negative thoughts from your mind.

Going with the flow: Enjoying yoga

Yoga is a form of exercise that combines physical ability with mind relaxation. Enjoying yoga on a regular basis can make you feel not only physically better but emotionally stronger, as well.

Most Westernized yoga focuses on the physical poses of yoga, or the *asanas*. These asanas stretch your muscles and help release the buildup of lactic acids, which cause fatigue, pain, and tension. One of the biggest benefits of yoga is its effect on the heart: By lowering blood pressure and slowing the heart rate, yoga can help prevent various kinds of heart disease and heart attacks. It also helps alleviate back pain and symptoms of asthma.

You can find a variety of yoga poses and levels of complexity, so feel free to experiment until you find moves that work best for you. Here are the two types of poses we introduce in this section:

- ✔ **Seated yoga poses:** Seated poses are good for grounding and centering, and they're good for getting started because they "open" the muscles for more movement later; these poses include the Butterfly, Lotus, and One Leg Forward Bend.

- ✔ **Standing yoga poses:** Standing poses are energetic and great for building strength and balance; they include Downward Dog, Tree, and Eagle.

For more yoga poses, you can check out *Yoga For Dummies,* 2nd Edition, by Georg Feuerstein and Larry Payne (John Wiley & Sons, Inc.) or the DVD *Basic Yoga Workout For Dummies* (Starz Entertainment).

Butterfly

Sit on your mat with your back straight. Bring your feet together and bend your knees, lifting your knees slightly off the ground. Hold your feet or ankles.

Lotus

The Lotus is probably one of the more well-known yoga positions. Sit cross-legged on your mat with your back straight. Slowly place your left foot onto your right thigh, and then place your right foot onto your left thigh. Rest your hands on your knees.

One Leg Forward Bend

Sit with your knees to your chest. Slowly stretch one leg out straight, while bending the other leg, allowing the knee to fall off to the side and with your foot making contact with your inner thigh. Hold for 20 seconds and then switch.

Downward Dog

Start on your hands and knees. Make sure your shoulders are over your wrists and your knees are hip-distance apart. Lift your hips up and straighten your arms and legs, extending your body into a high upside-down V shape. See Figure 19-3. *Note:* Straighten your legs only as far as is comfortable to you.

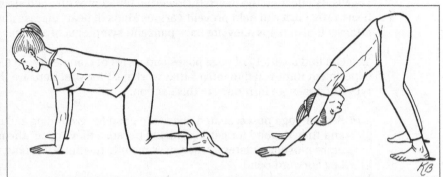

Figure 19-3:
Downward
Dog pose
strength-
ens your
shoulders
and upper
body while
stretching
your leg
muscles.

Tree

While standing, shift all your weight to one foot. Then lift the other foot and
place it on your standing leg — on your inner thigh or as high as you're able
to place it, even if that's just on your calf. Lift your arms straight over your
head. See Figure 19-4.

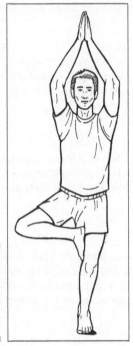

Figure 19-4:
Tree pose
requires
focus and
balance.

Eagle

Start in a standing position and shift all your weight to one foot. Bend your knee slightly and lift your other leg, wrapping it over and around your other leg. Hook the top of your foot around your calf. Wrap your arms in a twisted position in front of you. See Figure 19-5.

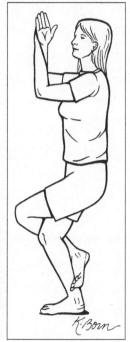

Figure 19-5:
Eagle pose helps you increase balance and strength.

Part V
The Part of Tens

The 5th Wave   By Rich Tennant

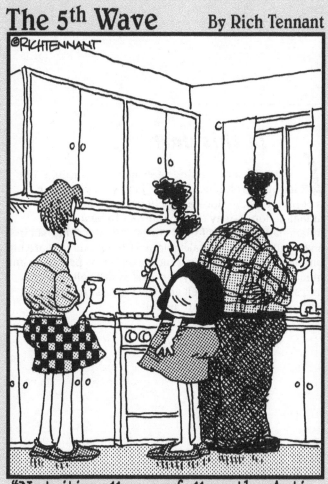

"Nutritionally, we follow the Anti-Inflammatory Food Guide Pyramid. When I first met Philip, he ate from the Food Guide Stonehenge. It was a mysterious diet, and no one's sure what its purpose was."

In this part . . .

*L*ike the idea of keeping a few lists at your fingertips
for quick reference? That's just what you get in
this part. First, we look at ten benefits of stopping
inflammation — why using your diet to beat down
inflammation both before it starts and after it has set in is
a good idea. Next, we take a look at ten foods that are high
on the list of those you should be eating as part of an anti-
inflammatory diet. Finally, we look at drug alternatives
and supplements and tell you the ten best to use along
with your anti-inflammation diet.

Chapter 20

Ten Benefits of Stopping Inflammation in Its Tracks

*Y*ou know lowering inflammation can make you feel less bad, but did you know that anti-inflammatory foods can actually make you feel *good?* Eating right and getting rid of the pain and irritation of inflammation can elevate your mood, which in turn makes you want to move more, socialize more, and just do more. Without achy joints, you may be more willing to take that walk with a friend. Without irritable bowel syndrome, you may be less afraid to try that new restaurant down the street. And without C-reactive protein (CRP) working against you, you may feel more like finishing that crossword puzzle, taking a stroll down memory lane, or just relaxing with the family.

This chapter highlights ten benefits of combating inflammation with changes to your diet (among other strategies covered in this book). We're sure you'll find more benefits than what we share here, but these are some that we find the most motivating.

Making You Feel Happier

Inflammation can make you just feel crummy. You're tired, your legs hurt, your arms hurt. You're not sleeping well and have an increased risk for cancer or heart disease. It's no wonder inflammation can put you in a bad mood. But decreasing inflammation doesn't just get rid of all those reasons to feel bad; it also has a positive effect on your brain chemistry.

You've heard the sayings about "an apple a day keeps the doctor away" or "all anyone needs is chocolate" to make them feel better. There's more truth to that than you may think. Following an anti-inflammatory diet to reduce inflammation and lower risks for a number of chronic diseases also elevates the release of good *neurotransmitters,* the chemical signals in your brain. In other words, it makes you happy. People suffering from depression tend to have higher levels of inflammatory chemicals in their blood as well as a higher stress-induced inflammatory response. The omega-3 fatty acids found in fish, flax, and walnuts may be part of the anti-inflammatory response your brain gives, releasing neurotransmitters. Those neurotransmitters make you feel happier than they would if you didn't get them in your diet or supplements on a regular basis; without the omega-3 fatty acids enhancing those neurotransmitters, getting healthy may take quite a bit longer.

Inflammation affects your brain's ability to make "feel good" neurotransmitters. Eating foods high in nutrient-dense proteins, the precursors to the amino acids that make neurotransmitters, and omega-3 fatty acids allows your brain to produce the neurotransmitters that make you feel good and that reduce inflammation. Eating junk food has the opposite effect — it creates inflammation and takes up calories that could be better spent on brain-healthy food.

Decreasing stress and anger can do more than make you feel good. A 2004 Duke University study showed that men with more anger, depression, and hostility had higher levels of systemic inflammation, which also leads to increased risk of heart attacks and heart disease. Researchers studied U.S. veterans of the Vietnam War over a 10-year period and discovered that otherwise healthy men who are prone to anger, hostility, and depression produce higher levels of inflammation markers present in heart disease and stroke.

There are some easy ways to combat mood swings: Take a walk outside, particularly on a sunny day. You'll get an added dose of vitamin D and the sun will likely help boost your mood, as well. No sunshine? Get out the yoga mat and do a quick 15-minute workout or some yoga (see Chapter 19 for a guide to some simple yoga poses).

Staying Sharp

The inflammation signal C-reactive protein (CRP), which is linked to heart and cardiovascular disease, also interferes with cognitive function in children and adults and is linked to the development of Alzheimer's disease.

Following an anti-inflammatory diet doesn't have to start later in life; in fact, a 2007 University of Louisville study showed that high CRP levels cause cognitive dysfunction in school-aged children — and one way to lower those levels is to follow an anti-inflammatory diet. High-sensitivity C-reactive protein was linked to children with sleep-disordered breathing, such as sleep apnea and snoring. Those issues then contributed to the children exhibiting deficiencies in attention, problem solving, intelligence, and long- and short-term memory.

Curbing these issues with an anti-inflammatory diet early in life will not only decrease the risk of inflammatory problems later but also give the children an early start on a healthy lifestyle.

The brain benefits continue as you age: A 2007 Harvard study found that chronic low-level inflammation increases the risk of developing Alzheimer's disease, and having high levels of inflammatory markers in your blood may increase your risk by as much as 250 percent.

Lowering Your Risk of Heart and Cardiovascular Disease

Inflammation, not simply the high cholesterol levels that have been blamed for so long, is an initiator of heart disease. In fact, cholesterol is just your body's way of trying to patch up the damage caused by inflammation.

A blood test called the hsCRP (highly sensitive cardio C-reactive protein) measures how much of this inflammatory substance is being produced in your body and rates it according to your risk of developing cardiovascular disease. If you have an elevated hsCRP, you can decrease your risk (and your inflammation numbers) by following an anti-inflammatory diet.

To make the diet more specific for you, consult with a physician trained in identifying and addressing food allergies and sensitivities in order to identify which foods to avoid. The physician can also guide you in ways to follow an anti-inflammatory diet and lifestyle that's tailored to your needs.

Decreasing Your Cholesterol Levels

High cholesterol may not be the cause of cardiovascular disease, but it's still a pretty meaningful risk factor. By following an anti-inflammatory diet and lifestyle, you can decrease your cholesterol because you're removing foods from your diet that increase blood cholesterol and triglyceride levels (that also happen to increase inflammation), such as saturated fat, inflammatory protein sources, fried foods, and cured meats. You're also increasing foods that decrease cholesterol (and inflammation), such as fresh vegetables, fruit, legumes, and whole grains.

In a 2005 study, researchers at Penn State University found that reducing dietary cholesterol was effective in reducing heart disease only in people with a low level of inflammation, as measured by CRP levels, and that people in the study with high CRP levels actually had an increase in their cholesterol levels while following a standard cholesterol-lowering diet. The researchers concluded that not only does decreasing inflammation reduce your risk of heart and cardiovascular disease, but it's also the best way to make a cholesterol-reducing diet beneficial.

Decreasing Your Risk of Diabetes and Metabolic Syndrome

High insulin levels are associated with insulin resistance and a diminished ability for the cells to take in glucose, and are a sign and precursor to diabetes, called *prediabetes*. Inflammation caused by high insulin levels makes the whole process get worse. Both high insulin and high glucose make the cells less responsive, and inflammation increases the risk of developing insulin resistance and glucose dysregulation.

In a 2007 study, researchers at the University of California-San Diego School of Medicine discovered that inflammation provoked by immune cells called *macrophages* led to insulin resistance and Type 2 diabetes. Inflammation and high insulin and blood glucose levels are a two-way street. The best way to decrease your risk of diabetes, prediabetes, and metabolic syndrome is to reduce inflammation and get your blood sugar under control.

Getting your blood sugar and insulin levels under control involves following an anti-inflammatory diet and remembering how quickly a food turns into sugar in your body, as measured by the glycemic load (GL) of foods. According to the *American Journal of Clinical Nutrition,* a 2002 review of studies on glycemic index and glycemic load on developing Type 2 diabetes confirmed that the glycemic load of carbohydrates affects inflammatory response, with a lower-glycemic diet seeming to effectively reduce inflammation.

Losing Weight

Eating foods that cause inflammation can make you gain weight. Simply removing the "bad" foods that contribute to inflammation may lead to weight loss. Toxins accumulate in your fat cells, making it harder for those cells to provide chemical signals to the rest of your body regarding metabolism and endocrine function. By reducing inflammation, you're making sure that all your cells, including the fat cells, have the right membrane coating and are creating healthier signals for your body.

The chemical signals help with weight stabilization and let your body function at its best. The endocrine system regulates weight and hormones, influences risk of metabolic syndrome and diabetes, and more. When toxins accumulate in fat cells, they prevent the endocrine system from working correctly.

Obesity and inflammation go hand-in-hand. A collaborative study in 2007 by Longitudinal Studies Section, National Institute on Aging, National Institutes of Health, and Tuscany Region Health Agency showed that obesity promotes inflammation, and by losing weight on an anti-inflammatory diet, you can stop the vicious cycle from both ends.

Strengthening Your Bones

Decreasing inflammation with the right types of anti-inflammatory food choices increases your bone strength and helps prevent osteoporosis, the thinning of bone tissue and loss of bone density, and *osteopenia,* which is lower-than-normal bone mineral density.

Search for foods with strong concentrations of *phytonutrients* — plant-based antioxidants that go to battle with the free radicals that kick off a variety of illnesses, including osteoporosis. Examples of phytonutrients include beta-carotene and lycopene.

Decreasing Your Risk of Autoimmune Disorders

Inflammation plays a major role in the development and onset of *autoimmune disorders* — disorders that occur when the immune system goes into hyperat-tack mode and destroys healthy tissue. Examples of autoimmune disorders are rheumatoid arthritis, multiple sclerosis, lupus, Addison's disease, Grave's disease, and celiac disease.

It makes sense that decreasing your risk of inflammation would also decrease your risk of developing those disorders. Identifying and addressing the dietary causes of inflammation that are contributing to the autoimmune response helps stop the inflammatory fire and decreases symptoms naturally.

Researchers at the University of Manchester Medical School in England found that people who followed a diet rich in dietary *carotenoids* — the antioxidants that give fruits and vegetables their orange and yellow coloring — dramatically reduced their risk of rheumatoid arthritis.

A 2002 study at the Center for Genetics, Nutrition, and Health showed that omega-3 fatty acids, the fats found in fish and flaxseed, have also been shown to lower the risks of autoimmune disorders, particularly rheumatoid arthritis and multiple sclerosis.

Affecting Risk and Ability to Fight Cancer

Multiple studies have shown that eating foods such as vegetables, fruits, and whole grains and that avoiding others, such as red meat and bad fats, lower cancer risk. But an anti-inflammation diet doesn't just lower your cancer risk; it can also help people who already have cancer.

Inflammation creates a state of chaos rather than calm for damaged or sick cells, especially cancer cells. Instead of attacking and killing the diseased cells, inflammation provides a "healing ground" for them, allowing them to not only grow but multiply. Maintaining a healthy diet of anti-inflammatory foods can help keep inflammation in check and the immune system working efficiently.

Improving Fertility

Infertility is on the rise for both men and women. Fertility is highest when inflammation is low or nonexistent, and keeping inflammation down can lower the risk of pre-eclampsia and miscarriage during pregnancy. Decreasing inflammation with antioxidants and omega-3 fish oils has been shown to improve fertility and decrease complications of pregnancy.

Pre-eclampsia is a condition in which the woman's blood pressure is elevated, posing a threat to both mother and child. Blood samples from women with pre-eclampsia were analyzed in a 1998 study from the Center for Perinatoa Studies in Seattle and were found to have lower omega-3 fatty acids and a higher omega-6-to-omega-3 fatty acid ratio.

A 2002 study from the Schwartz Center for Metabolism and Nutrition at Case Western University showed that improving blood insulin and glucose regulation through an anti-inflammatory diet is effective in reducing incidence of polycystic ovarian syndrome (PCOS), a disorder characterized by hormonal abnormalities, insulin resistance, abnormal cholesterol levels, and obesity. PCOS has been linked to infertility and increased inflammation.

Chapter 21

Ten Inflammation-Fighting Foods

In This Chapter

▶ Packing an anti-inflammatory punch into every meal

▶ Finding the medicinal properties of some foods

▶ Making green tea a go-to beverage

*Y*ou don't have to go any farther than your kitchen to start your fight against inflammation. Food can be just as powerful as medication in decreasing inflammation and reducing your risk of chronic disease. This chapter highlights ten of our favorite inflammation-fighting foods. Make them part of an anti-inflammatory diet, and the punch becomes much more powerful.

Salmon

Salmon is a great source of protein to work into main menus for breakfast, lunch, or dinner. It's an essential ingredient in anti-inflammatory diets because it contains high amounts of omega-3 fatty acids and has a multitude of health benefits: It can help reduce the risk of heart and cardiovascular disease; decrease triglycerides and lower blood pressure; prevent stroke and heart arrhythmias; and help with weight loss by improving *satiety,* or that feeling of fullness. It improves the body's ability to respond to insulin for better blood sugar control, reduces inflammation in autoimmune disorders, reduces cancer risk, and improves outcomes in some types of cancer, such as breast and colorectal cancers.

Omega-3s — and salmon, in particular — protect against macular degeneration (a disease that destroys sharp, central vision through the degeneration of the macula in retina) and dry eyes, help lubricate joints in arthritis, improve skin health for acne and dry skin, reduce the risk of asthma, improve cognition and mood, and reduce your risk for dementia and Alzheimer's disease.

Salmon contains two types of omega-3s — eicosapentaenoic acid (EPA) and docosahexaenoic acid (DHA) — but EPA is the primary one. EPA is a precursor to anti-inflammatory signals called *prostaglandins.* They prevent cardiovascular disease and improve blood flow. Salmon helps reduce inflammation for bone, joint, and muscle disorders by using EPA to produce compounds called *resolvins.* The resolvins prevent inflammatory cells and chemical signals from forming in the body.

In addition to the protein and omega-3 fatty acids, salmon contains high levels of vitamin D, selenium, niacin (vitamin B3), vitamin B12, phosphorus, and magnesium. A 4-ounce serving of salmon contains 87.1 percent of the recommended daily value for omega-3 fatty acids.

Eating at least two to three servings a week of salmon can give you as much EPA and DHA as most fish oil capsules. We recommend taking daily fish oil capsules or eating salmon at least three times a week. In general, you'll get better benefits with wild rather than farm-raised salmon. A study by the Environmental Working Group, a consumer protection agency, found that farmed salmon has 16 times the toxic polychlorinated biphenyls (PCBs) than wild salmon does.

You can serve *lox,* which is cured salmon, on gluten-free bread for breakfast. A piece of steamed salmon on a hearty green salad and salmon steaks for dinner round out a full menu of this healthy fish. You have plenty of ways to cook salmon, too — it can be broiled, steamed, baked, cured with lemon juice, and added to pates.

Flaxseeds

Flaxseeds are tiny brown seeds of *Linum usitatissium,* a plant that people have used as a source of food, fiber for clothing, and medicine for centuries.

The anti-inflammatory benefits in flaxseeds come from their high amounts of an omega-3 fatty acid, *alpha linolenic acid* (ALA), which is a precursor to the anti-inflammatory compound EPA, which we discuss in the preceding section.

Flaxseeds help improve bone health by preventing excessive bone turnover (a change in the balance between bone loss and bone formation), protect against heart disease and diabetes, and help improve blood sugar control. A study of patients with high cholesterol found that eating 20 grams of ground flaxseed daily significantly reduced levels of total cholesterol, LDL cholesterol (the bad kind), triglycerides, and the ratio of total to HDL cholesterol after 60 days.

The phytoestrogens in flaxseeds balance the body's hormone levels by acting as selective estrogen response modifiers (SERM), a similar mechanism to the popular breast cancer drug tamoxifen. When estrogen is low, SERMs weakly bind to estrogen sites to boost estrogen, and when estrogen is high, SERMs take up the space of estrogen receptors to reduce heightened estrogen levels. The phytoestrogen activity in flaxseeds has been found to be protective against breast cancer.

Besides omega-3 fatty acids, lignans, and dietary fiber, flaxseeds are high in the nutrients manganese, folate, copper, phosphorus, and vitamin B6. A tablespoon of ground flaxseeds contains approximately 1.8 grams of omega-3 fatty acids, which is good for your body.

 Between 1 to 2 tablespoons of ground flaxseed a day are helpful for hormone, blood sugar, and anti-inflammatory balance. Studies have shown that 4 tablespoons daily can significantly reduce blood cholesterol levels. If you're introducing flaxseed into your diet, you should start with small amounts and work up to 1 to 2 tablespoons per day.

For the full fiber effect you should consume whole flaxseeds, but all the other nutrients are present in ground flaxseed as well. *Note:* Keep whole flaxseed on hand and grind it as needed; ground flaxseed has a short shelf life.

Although flaxseeds do have a slightly nutty taste, most people don't detect a taste at all. You can easily add them to shakes, yogurt (if you can tolerate dairy), salads, or baked goods or use them as a nut substitute without compromising taste. Because of their high fiber content, flaxseeds and ground flax have a mealy consistency and may make a yogurt shake or oatmeal thicker. Flaxseeds are gluten-free, so you can add them to gluten-free recipes and use them along with gluten-free flours.

Blueberries

Blueberries are high in *antioxidants* (specifically flavonoids and anthocyandins), which protect cells from inflammation and oxidative stress. The anthocyandins, which give blueberries their blue-red color, help keep blood vessels and capillaries strong, stabilize the "glue" of your body called *collagen* (the stuff that binds cells together), help stop the proliferation of cancer, and enhance the antioxidant effects of vitamin C. Blueberries also contain fiber, manganese, and vitamins C, E, and K.

Blueberries improve night vision and protect against macular degeneration, prevent aging of the brain due to free-radical damage, prevent dementia, improve learning and motor skills, and provide cancer protection through antioxidants called *ellagic acid*. Blueberries also protect against colon and ovarian cancer, help lower cholesterol, and reduce the risk of urinary tract infections. These delicious, versatile berries even have a low glycemic index, which makes them a good choice for people with blood sugar issues.

Any amount of blueberries is good to eat on a daily or weekly basis. One cup of blueberries every day provides approximately 20 percent of the daily value of manganese and 10 percent of the daily recommendation of vitamin E. Aim for incorporating at least a cup into your diet three times a week. Eat fresh blueberries for dessert, or add them to yogurt, oatmeal, smoothies, salads, or whole grain pancakes.

Natural Almonds

Once frowned upon as a high-fat snack, almonds are now touted as one of the top superfoods you should include in your diet, particularly in an anti-inflammatory diet.

The monounsaturated fat, protein, and potassium in natural almonds make them good promoters of heart health, and the vitamin E they contain is an antioxidant and helps prevent heart attacks. Almonds also help temper the rise in insulin and blood sugar, helping to fight diabetes. And almonds are a good source of folic acid, which helps prevent birth defects.

Almonds have about 6 grams of protein in a 1-ounce serving, which is a small handful. They're stuffed with vitamins and minerals: thiamin, riboflavin, niacin, biotin, and vitamin E. In fact, one serving of almonds has 40 percent of your daily recommended value of vitamin E.

Mushrooms

Mushrooms belong to an enigmatic class of fungus that grows in the dark woods and thrives on rainy, moist days. Edible mushrooms are also one of the most immune-boosting, nutrient-packed, and anti-inflammatory foods you can include in your diet. They contain high amounts of antioxidants, phyto-nutrients, and sugars called *polysaccharides,* which regulate the immune system.

The list of benefits from mushrooms is long, as is the list of nutrients you find in them. One of the most cited health benefits of mushrooms is helping the immune system's white blood cells protect your body against infection, cardiovascular disease, cancer, and arthritis. Mushrooms, especially maitake mushrooms, help regulate blood sugar in diabetes. Mushrooms also provide potent antioxidant protection; shiitake, maitake, and reishi mushrooms have anti-cancer effects, and white button mushrooms may also protect against breast and prostate cancer. And if that weren't enough, mushrooms also help to increase ovulation in women suffering from polycystic ovarian syndrome (PCOS).

Mushrooms contain 10 percent of your daily value of protein and 5 percent of your fiber in just a 5-ounce serving. Five ounces of crimini mushrooms contain more than 50 percent of the recommended daily value of selenium. In addition, mushrooms contain high amounts of vitamin B2, copper, vitamin B3, tryptophan, vitamin B5, potassium, phosphorus, zinc, manganese, vitamin B1, vitamin B6, folate, magnesium, iron, and calcium.

Mushrooms come in many varieties and shapes. You can eat them raw, cooked, or dehydrated in salads, soups, side dishes, stews, and main courses. A half-cup of mushrooms daily gives you half your daily requirements of the antioxidant selenium as well as other anti-inflammatory and immune system-boosting benefits.

Broccoli

Broccoli is one of those superfoods you can eat in a variety of ways — raw, steamed, in soups and salads — and it still maintains a high level of nutrients and nourishment.

The dietary fiber in broccoli can help keep your intestines clean, and the calcium and iron promote strong bones and red blood cells. Broccoli also helps protect against heart disease, some cancers, and diabetes.

In just one medium stalk of broccoli, you can get 12 percent of your daily fiber needs and 3 percent of your daily carbohydrates. And the more broccoli you eat, the better off you are. Broccoli is also full of vitamins C and D, calcium, iron, folate, and phytonutrients.

Quinoa

Quinoa is on the anti-inflammatory list because it's a whole grain that's also a *complete protein,* which means it contains all the essential amino acids — you don't need to eat it with other legumes to get its protein benefit. Even though quinoa is a whole grain, quinoa is actually related to the spinach and beet family. It's gluten-free and safe for people with celiac disease.

Studies have shown that quinoa prevents migraine headaches because it's high in magnesium and riboflavin (vitamin B2), which help reduce inflammation in the blood vessels. Including whole grains like quinoa in the diet can also protect you against heart and cardiovascular disease, asthma, gallstones, Type 2 diabetes, and cancer.

Just 3.5 ounces of cooked quinoa contain 14 grams of protein and 7 grams of dietary fiber. Quinoa is high in manganese, magnesium, iron, tryptophan, copper, and phosphorus.

Use quinoa as a substitute for other carbohydrates or starches in the diet, such as pasta or rice, or use quinoa flour as a gluten-free flour substitute. (Always remember to rinse quinoa before cooking it.) We recommend eating 1 cup of quinoa at least three to five times a week as part of the healthy whole-grain portion of your diet.

Brussels Sprouts

Brussels sprouts are a hearty cruciferous vegetable that's high in antioxidant and antioxidant nutrients, including vitamin K. Surprisingly enough, they also contain *alpha-linolenic acid,* the omega-3, anti-inflammatory fatty acid found in salmon and flaxseeds (read up on salmon and flax earlier in the chapter).

Brussels sprouts aid in detoxification because they contain compounds called *glucosinolates,* which are necessary for enzymes of detoxification that aid in the fight against and possible prevention of some cancers. Brussels sprouts can also help reduce the risk of cardiovascular disease, decrease cholesterol, aid in digestion and bowel regularity, and thwart *Helicobacter pylori,* the bacterium that causes peptic ulcer disease.

One cup of steamed Brussels sprouts has 15 percent of the daily recommended value of fiber, 10 percent of the daily value of protein, and about 12 percent of the omega-3 fatty acids you need. They're high in vitamins K, C, A, B6, B1, B2, and E as well as folate, manganese, potassium, tryptophan, iron, phosphorus, magnesium, copper, and calcium.

Add Brussels sprouts to soups or salads, steam them, boil them, or bake them and add them to your main meals. Add 1 cup of Brussels sprouts to your dietary regime two to three times a week or more to get the positive detoxification benefits.

Onions

Onions provide a powerhouse of anti-inflammatory benefits and are easy to incorporate into most meals. They're high in sulfur-containing molecules that your body's cells need to function properly. The sulfur molecules also help keep your joints lubricated, which means onions support healthy bone and connective tissue.

Onions also aid in detoxification and boost immune function. They protect against cardiovascular disease; protect against colorectal, laryngeal, and ovarian cancers; and improve blood-sugar control in diabetics.

Onions are high in chromium, vitamins C and B6, manganese, molybdenum, tryptophan, folate, potassium, phosphorus, and copper. A half cup of onions contains approximately 100 milligrams of the antioxidant and anti-inflammatory flavonoid *quercetin.*

Use onions raw in sandwiches or add them to soups and salads. Chop up and sauté onions in olive oil and add them to omelets, fish, poultry, beans — just about *anything.* Incorporate at least a half a cup of onions daily in your diet.

Green Tea

Green tea comes in many varieties and flavors and is one of the most anti-inflammatory beverages you can drink, other than water. It contains high amounts of the antioxidant compounds (called *catechins*) and circulatory stimulants (called *theobromide* and *theophylline*).

Other teas, such as white, black, and oolong, are extremely healthy as well, but when it comes to listing the ten best "superfoods," green tea is a real standout.

Epigallocatechin-3-gallate, or EGCG, is the catechin that people believe is responsible for tea's anticancer benefits. Researchers have studied it extensively for its health properties. Green tea catechins may also prevent *angiogenesis,* which is the formation of blood vessels that provide access to "food" to cancer cells.

Regular drinkers of green tea have lower rates of heart disease and low-ered risk of developing various cancers. In addition, green tea improves insulin insensitivity, reduces the risk of eye disease, and reduces the anti-stress effects due to the L-theanine and neuroprotection in Alzheimer's and Parkinson's diseases.

Drink at least one to three 6-ounce cups of green tea a day to get its antioxi-dant and anti-inflammatory benefits.

If you're on a blood thinner such as *Coumadin* or *warfarin,* consult your phy-sician before consuming large amounts of green tea. Tea may increase the effects of these blood-thinning medications due its anti-platelet and anticoagu-lant activity, making it less likely for platelets to stick together and form clots.

Chapter 22

Ten Anti-Inflammatory Supplements and Herbs

....

In This Chapter

▶ Discovering how supplements work to decrease inflammation

▶ Knowing how to choose the best supplements

▶ Understanding risks of anti-inflammatory supplements

....

C hanging your diet to include anti-inflammatory foods, spices, herbs, and beverages is the first and most important step in the battle against inflammation and chronic disease. Getting a lot of good exercise — both heart-pumping cardiovascular workouts and relaxing yoga — is another good step.

Finding those supplements — natural herbs and enzymes — that give your new diet that extra boost is an added bonus in the fight against inflammation. From herbs that keep migraines at bay to vitamins that help reduce the risk of cancer, supplements should be part of your daily routine. We discuss our top ten anti-inflammatory herb and supplement picks in this chapter. Read on for info on the benefits, the recommended dosages, and the cautions and contraindications associated with these supplements.

Always consult a physician or pharmacist who is knowledgeable in herbs and supplements and their interactions before trying any herbs or supplements on your own.

Omega-3 Fatty Acids: Mixed EPA and DHA from Fish Oils

Eicosapentaenoic acid (EPA) and docosahexaenoic acid (DHA) are two essential fatty acids derived from fish and some vegetarian sources. You can't make these fatty acids in your body — that's why they're essential fatty acids — so you need to get them from food or supplements daily. EPA and DHA are anti-inflammatory superstars because they compete against a pro-inflammatory compound called arachidonic acid (AA) for incorporation into cellular membranes.

Use fish (such as salmon and sardines) and fish oils as your primary sources of EPA and DHA. Vegetarian sources of omega-3 fatty acids (flax and chia, for example) contain *alpha linolenic acid* (ALA), which gets converted into EPA.

If you can't find fish that are low in mercury and other toxins, take a high-quality fish oil supplement with both EPA and DHA for an anti-inflammatory diet.

Just as important as the positives that take place when you do supplement your diet with fish oils is what happens when you don't: Some studies have linked an omega-3 deficiency to an increased risk of depression.

Here are some basic ideas you should know about increasing your intake of mixed EPA and DHA from fish oils:

- ✔ **Checking for quality:** Choose fish oil supplements that are good manufacturing practice (GMP)-certified and tested for heavy metals. They should smell like fresh fish when you bite into a capsule. Quality fish oils cost a little more than other brands and have been tested for shelf stability.
- ✔ **Dosing:** Take 1 to 4 grams daily of a mixed EPA/DHA.
- ✔ **Cautions/contraindications:** Because fish oils have benefits similar to blood thinners, they may increase the effect of pharmaceutical blood thinners, such as warfarin (Coumadin).

Ginger

The root of the ginger plant has increased in popularity in recent years, and no wonder — it has multiple anti-inflammatory benefits and helps reduce symptoms in inflammatory disorders. Among the benefits of ginger, and more specifically gingerroot, are the following:

- ✔ It decreases inflammation by inhibiting the cyclooxygenase and lipoxygenase pathways, prostaglandin E2, thromboxane B2, and tumor necrosis factor (TNF-alpha).
- ✔ It decreases pain in disorders such as osteoarthritis and rheumatoid arthritis.
- ✔ It's antibacterial and antifungal.

✔ It decreases fevers.

✔ It aids with nausea, including the nausea of pregnancy and the nausea and vomiting of chemotherapy.

✔ It decreases the risk of heart and cardiovascular disease by increasing circulation and preventing the clotting of blood.

✔ It may be used as a prophylactic for migraine headaches.

Here are some basic facts you should know about taking ginger:

✔ **Checking for quality:** Fresh is always best, but you can use dried ginger or encapsulated ginger extracts.

✔ **Dosing:** 1 to 2 grams of fresh or dried ginger a day can help with pain, aches, and inflammation. Drink 1 to 3 cups of ginger tea for aches and pains or add a ¼-inch piece of peeled, diced ginger to your stir-fry. Capsules containing at least 170 milligrams of gingerroot extract, taken three times a day, are helpful with arthritis.

✔ **Caution/contraindications:** Ginger may interact with blood thinners like warfarin (Coumadin), so consult your physician before adding it to your diet in large amounts. People with gallstones or those who have experienced a peptic ulcer should take caution in taking ginger, as should anyone taking antacids.

Turmeric/Curcumin

Turmeric comes from the root of the Indian *Curcuma longa* plant and is a main ingredient in curry. It contains an extract called *curcumin* that researchers have studied extensively for its multiple anti-inflammatory benefits. Curcumin lends the spice its bright orange color.

Curcumin works in much the same way as ibuprofen but without the gastrointestinal side effects. That is, it inhibits the inflammatory cascade (the competition of different cells for the same enzyme) in the body mediated by cyclooxygenase-2 (COX-2), prostaglandins, and leukotrienes. Curcumin also works as an antioxidant and stimulates the immune system.

Here are some of the anti-inflammatory benefits of curcumin:

✔ It helps relieve indigestion by increasing digestive enzymes.

✔ It has hepatoprotective effects, which protect against liver damage.

✔ It helps with cognitive function and may decrease the risk of dementia and Alzheimer's disease.

✔ It reduces the pain and inflammation symptoms of rheumatoid arthritis.

✔ It works as a cancer preventative by inhibiting tumor promotion, inhibiting the growth of cancer cells, and reducing their blood supply.

✔ It may help with circulation by preventing the platelets from clumping together.

Here are some basic facts you should know about taking curcumin:

✔ **Checking for quality:** The price of a curcumin extract may reflect its quality and standardization. The better-quality companies ensure that they have a good quality of turmeric to start and have the right amount of curcumin in each bottle, so quality extracts cost a bit more.

✔ **Dosing:** For anti-inflammatory benefit, you may need to take 500 milligrams up to three times a day. Turmeric and curcumin seem to be better absorbed with food.

✔ **Caution/contraindications:** Curcumin should not be taken by people with gallstones or obstructed bile ducts without first consulting a physician. It can increase risk of serious bleeding, so it shouldn't be taken by people with bleeding disorders or those who are taking blood thinning medication.

NAC (N-acetyl cysteine)

N-acetyl cysteine (NAC) is a derivative of amino acids, the building blocks of protein. NAC reduces free-radical damage and stops inflammation by acting as an antioxidant.

Here are some of the anti-inflammatory benefits of NAC:

✔ It protects against drug toxicity and aspirin poisoning.

✔ It promotes liver detoxification.

✔ It helps lower the risk of cardiovascular disease by decreasing homocysteine.

✔ It prevents bronchitis and improves the condition of people with chronic obstructive pulmonary disease (COPD).

✔ It's a cancer protective.

✔ It increases circulation by preventing platelet aggregation.

✔ It helps protect the immune system in HIV disease.

✔ It helps relieve compulsive psychiatric disorders.

Here are some basic facts you should know about taking NAC:

- ✔ **Checking for quality:** Make sure you get your supplements from a reputable source or a doctor who specializes in nutritional supplements.

- ✔ **Dosing:** A general safe dose is 600 milligrams once or twice a day. Always consult your physician before starting any new herbs or supplements.

- ✔ **Caution/contraindications:** NAC is generally safe, although people taking blood pressure medications, diabetes medications, and anticoagulants should avoid NAC due to some gastrointestinal side effects. Pregnant women should also avoid taking NAC.

Bromelain

Bromelain, an enzyme derived from pineapple, decreases the inflammatory response of the immune system and works as an antioxidant to increase reactive oxygen species (ROS) that clean up the mess of inflammation.

Bromelain also helps with circulation by inhibiting platelet aggregation, and it works against cancer by disrupting the growth of cancer cells. A study in osteoarthritis of the knee showed that a combination of bromelain with other antioxidants at 50 milligrams three times a day worked as well as the medication diclofenac (Voltaren) in reducing pain and improving function.

Here are some other anti-inflammatory benefits of bromelain:

- ✔ It aids in digestion.
- ✔ It helps with healing after surgery and trauma.
- ✔ It helps alleviate allergy symptoms.
- ✔ It eases aches and pains by acting as a smooth muscle relaxant, and it reduces muscle soreness after workouts.
- ✔ It has cardiovascular and circulatory applications, including the inhibition of thrombus formation and platelet aggregation.
- ✔ It helps reduce the inflammatory symptoms of inflammatory bowel diseases such as ulcerative colitis.

Here are some basic facts you should know about taking bromelain:

- ✔ **Checking for quality:** Make sure you get your supplements from a reputable source or a doctor who specializes in nutritional supplements.

- ✔ **Dosing:** 200 to 1,000 milligrams a day is generally used for arthritis and pain. It should be taken in divided doses on an empty stomach.

✔ **Caution/contraindications:** Because bromelain has anti-platelet aggregation activity, you should use it with caution alongside other medications that work the same way, such as warfarin (Coumadin) and other blood thinners. Those with allergies to pineapple should avoid this supplement.

Boswellia

Boswellia, the tree resin from the *Boswellia serrata* plant, is also called *Indian frankincense.* It contains boswellic acid and alpha and beta boswellic acid, which researchers found to have anti-inflammatory properties in laboratory research. The anti-inflammatory properties of the boswellic acids come from their ability to prevent the formation of chemical signals in the body for inflammation, namely 5 lipoxygenase, leukotrienes, and leukocyte elastase.

Boswellia is an arthritis pain reliever in that it decreases the breakdown of cartilage and helps keep the joints lubricated. For autoimmune disease, boswellia appears to inhibit the chemical signals of autoimmune disease and reduce the formation of *antibodies,* the body's attack cells.

Among boswellia's benefits are the following:

✔ It decreases inflammation in osteoarthritis, rheumatoid arthritis, tendonitis, bursitis, and general aches and pains.

✔ It's used to decrease inflammation in inflammatory bowel diseases such as ulcerative colitis and Crohn's disease.

✔ It may help decrease inflammation in asthma and allergies.

✔ It has antibacterial and antiviral properties.

✔ It has been shown to prevent cancer cell growth and help with programmed cancer cell death in colon cancer.

✔ It protects against certain autoimmune diseases and their symptoms.

Here are some basic facts you should know about taking boswellia:

✔ **Checking for quality:** Make sure you get your supplements from a reputable source or a doctor who specializes in nutritional supplements.

✔ **Dosing:** 300 milligrams three times a day is generally used for arthritis and inflammatory disorders.

✔ **Caution/contraindications:** Boswellia is generally safe.

Vitamin D

Vitamin D is probably one of the easiest nutrients to obtain, yet is one in which the majority of people have deficiencies. Vitamin D is a fat-soluble vitamin that is stimulated in the skin by exposure to the sun and is found in small amounts in some foods. A laboratory test called 25-hydroxy vitamin D shows that most people are vitamin D deficient unless they spend time outside in full sun every day.

The following are among vitamin D's many anti-inflammatory benefits:

- It boosts the immune system.

- It prevents *rickets,* a disorder causing bones to become weak and deformed.

- It protects against muscle aches and pains.

- It prevents osteoporosis and osteopenia and reduces the risk of bone fracture.

- It lowers the risk of autoimmune disorders such as rheumatoid arthritis and MS, and it improves symptoms in people with such disorders.

- It helps with blood sugar regulation, and it may prevent Type 1 diabetes.

- It protects against heart and cardiovascular disease. Researchers think vitamin D does this by affecting inflammatory mediators such as tumor necrosis factor-alpha (TNF-alpha) and interleukin.

- It decreases the risk of cancer, specifically breast, prostate, and colon cancers.

Here are some basic facts you should know about vitamin D:

- **Checking for quality:** Make sure to use vitamin D3 rather than vitamin D2.

- **Dosing:** In general, most adults need 1,000 to 4,000 IU (international units) of vitamin D daily. However, people with autoimmune disease and who are very deficient in the vitamin may need more to achieve optimal blood levels. We list some dietary sources of vitamin D3 in Table 22-1.

  Full-body sun exposure for about 12 minutes during the sunniest part of the day (midday) produces approximately 10,000 units of vitamin D. If you're unable to get this exposure, exposing the hands, face, arms, and legs to sunlight two to three times a week for about a quarter of the time it would take you to get a mild sunburn will cause the skin to produce minimal requirements of vitamin D. So if you normally start to turn pink after 20 minutes in the sun, try for 5 minutes of sun exposure two to three times a week; that could be as easy as walking to the end of your street and back. It's important to mention, however, that a variety of factors — clothing, sunscreen, dark skin pigmentation, and air pollution, among others — can limit the sun's strength and therefore the amount of vitamin D the body is stimulated to produce.

✔ **Caution/contraindications:** Toxicity due to too much vitamin D is rare; in fact, the only studies that showed toxicity used 100,000 IU or more given intravenously. You'd need 25-hydroxyvitamin D blood levels of 150 ng/mL or more to get toxicity from vitamin D.

Caution is advised with vitamin D in people with liver disease, people with high blood calcium levels, and people with granulomatous disorders such as sarcoidosis and tuberculosis (TB).

Table 22-1	Dietary Sources of Vitamin D3
Food	*Vitamin D per 100 g*
Cod liver oil	10,000 IU (up to 25,555 IU)
Herring	680 IU
Oysters	642 IU
Catfish	500 IU
Sardines	480 IU
Mackerel	450 IU
Salmon	320 IU
Caviar	232 IU
Shrimp	172 IU
Butter	56 IU
Whole egg (contained in yolk only)	49 IU
Most plant foods	0 IU

www.cholesterol-and-health.com/Vitamin-D.html

For more complete coverage of vitamin D, check out *Vitamin D For Dummies* by Alan L. Rubin, MD (John Wiley & Sons, Inc.).

Vitamin C

Vitamin C, also known as *ascorbic acid,* is a water-soluble vitamin that decreases inflammation by acting as a potent antioxidant. Vitamin C also decreases C-reactive protein, the protein that gets elevated when your body is inflamed.

You can find high amounts of vitamin C in vegetables and fruits, including broccoli, papaya, bell peppers, oranges, cantaloupe, kiwi, cauliflower, Brussels sprouts, and strawberries. Overcooking and prolonged storage decrease the vitamin C content in food, so eat these fruits and vegetables raw or slightly cooked.

Among the anti-inflammatory benefits of vitamin C are the following:

- It's an antioxidant.
- It stimulates the immune system and prevents infections.
- It helps decrease allergy symptoms.
- It prevents gout by decreasing uric acid levels.
- It helps people with cardiovascular disease by preventing free radical damage.
- It helps maintain connective tissue integrity to prevent wrinkles.
- It protects the skin against sun damage.
- It can be used adjunctively in cancer care or to help with cancer prevention (although consultation with an oncologist is necessary and appropriate).
- It prevents *scurvy,* a disease caused by a deficiency in vitamin C that includes the swelling and bleeding of the gums and the opening of previously healed wounds.
- It aids in wound healing.
- It may aid in increasing HDL (good) cholesterol.

Here are some basic facts you should know about increasing your intake of vitamin C:

- **Checking for quality:** Vitamin C can be made synthetically in a lab or derived from food sources, such as rose hips. Food-derived sources may be better absorbed than synthetic sources because the body can't absorb more than 1 gram at a time — the rest is lost through urine.

✔ **Dosing:** You need at least 100 milligrams a day to prevent scurvy and 1 to 3 grams a day for optimal function in preventing oxidative damage due to free radicals and increasing immune support. Start with 100 milligrams a day and slowly increase to 1 to 3 grams. The upper limit of vitamin C is determined by bowel tolerance (too much vitamin C will lead to loose stools). If you hit that upper limit, begin scaling back your daily amount of vitamin C.

✔ **Caution/contraindications:** Too much vitamin C causes diarrhea and stomach upset. It's safe in doses up to the point where it causes loose stools, called *bowel tolerance.* For adults, the recommended daily maximum of vitamin C is 2,000 milligrams.

Papain

Papain, an enzyme derived from the fruit of the papaya plant, helps reduce inflammation by breaking down harmful substances in the body and releasing substances such as reactive oxygen species (ROS) and cytokines that reduce inflammation and have antioxidant function.

Here are some of papain's anti-inflammatory benefits:

✔ It's a digestive aid/enzyme.

✔ It's used to help reduce inflammation and improve healing after surgery and trauma.

✔ It can help prevent post-operative adhesions.

✔ It can help reduce inflammation of the throat and may reduce symptoms of tonsillitis.

✔ It aids in wound healing.

✔ It may reduce pain and inflammation in rheumatic disease.

Here are some basic facts you should know about taking papain:

✔ **Checking for quality:** Make sure you get your supplements from a reputable source or a doctor who specializes in nutritional supplements.

✔ **Dosing:** 1,500 milligrams a day is the dose used to treat inflammation and swelling after surgery or trauma. Take it on an empty stomach for best results.

✔ **Caution/contraindications:** Some people may be allergic to papaya and papain. People with GERD and ulcers, as well as those taking immunosuppression therapy and radiation therapy, should be especially cautious when eating papain.

Coenzyme Q10

Coenzyme Q10 is a vitamin-like substance that provides energy to all the cells of your body. It's an antioxidant, and it helps stabilize the cell membranes. You need coenzyme Q10 to complete many of your metabolic functions. For example, the mitochondria in your cells use it to make adenosine triphosphate (ATP), your cells' main energy source.

Among the anti-inflammatory benefits of coenzyme Q10 are the following:

- ✔ It provides energy for all the cells of your body.
- ✔ It protects the heart and body against free-radical damage.
- ✔ It reduces the risk of heart disease and helps normalize blood pressure.
- ✔ It protects the body against muscle damage due to statin (cholesterol-lowering) drugs, such as Lipitor. Statins inhibit the enzyme needed to make cholesterol and coenzyme Q10.
- ✔ It may protect the brain against damage and aids in treating Parkinson's disease.
- ✔ It helps reduce the occurrence of migraine headaches.
- ✔ It has benefits in cancer protection.
- ✔ It helps protect the gums against gingivitis.

Here are some basic facts you should know about taking coenzyme Q10:

- ✔ **Checking for quality:** Coenzyme Q10 needs to be in an emulsified (fat-soluble) form in order to be absorbed. Some people who have difficulty absorbing coenzyme Q10 may do better with its derivative, called ubiquinol.
- ✔ **Dosing:** Generally, 60 to 100 milligrams a day provides good antioxidant protection.
- ✔ **Caution/contraindications:** Coenzyme Q10 looks like the blood thinning vitamin, vitamin K, so coenzyme Q10 may interact with other blood thinners. Have your physician monitor your blood if you're on a blood thinner such as warfarin (Coumadin).

Part VI
Appendixes

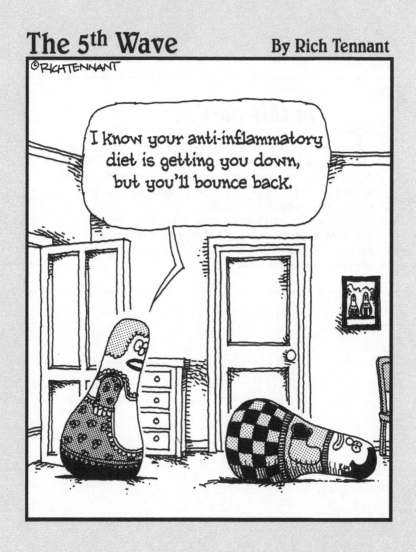

In this part . . .

The resources in this part are tools intended to help ease your transition to an anti-inflammatory lifestyle. Appendix A gives you background and information on the inflammation factor (IF) ratings system, a system that takes all the factors of certain foods — fats, sugars, carbohydrates, and more — and determines which are anti-inflammatory and which are pro-inflammatory. Appendix B is a metric unit conversion chart for people who use the metric system.

Appendix A

Inflammation Factor Ratings

● ●

*N*utritionist Monica Reinagel created the *inflammation factor* (IF) rating system with the intention of providing a way to predict the inflammatory effects of certain foods. Using a specialized formula, the IF ratings measure more than 20 elements of a food to determine its inflammatory or anti-inflammatory effects on the body. These elements include a food's amount and types of fat; the presence of vitamins, minerals, and anti-inflammatory compounds; and the food's *glycemic index,* a scale used to determine how fast and how high a food can raise the body's blood sugar (blood glucose) level.

By predicting how various foods affect the body, the IF rating system makes identifying inflammatory and anti-inflammatory foods easy. Foods with negative ratings are more likely to cause inflammation, and those with positive ratings are more likely to fight inflammation. The higher the number, the stronger the food is going to be in fighting inflammation.

Foods with a positive IF rating are those that contain anti-inflammatory nutrients, such as monounsaturated fats, folate, selenium, and docosahexaenoic acid (DHA). Foods with a negative IF rating are those with inflammatory nutrients, such as saturated fats and arachidonic acid, one of the main mechanisms for the development of pain and inflammation. In this section, we talk about balancing your total IF rating and finding the IF rating of individual foods.

Finding a balance

The goal isn't to avoid negative IF foods altogether. The main objective is to end the day with an overall positive IF rating, with a typical target of 50 (*Note:* Specific targets are available through Reinagel's program, which you can find online at www.inflammationfactor.com).

Say you want a breakfast of two hard-boiled eggs, a cup of blueberries, and an 8-ounce glass of apple juice. Sounds like a nice, healthy breakfast, right? Consider the numbers: The inflammation factor for each of the eggs is –51, so for two, it's –102; the IF rating for the blueberries is –28; and for the apple juice, it's –44. Everything you have in front of you is considered inflammatory on this scale, with a total IF rating of –174.

Does that mean you should skip that breakfast and move on to something else? Not at all. These foods contain nutrients that you need, such as antioxidants in the blueberries. You simply want to take foods with negative IF ratings in moderation.

Inflammation is a necessary and sometimes healthy process in the body, so it makes sense that a healthy diet would include some foods that support inflammatory responses. It's when the inflammatory response is excessive — when your total IF rating is in the negative — that it's not good.

Although you're starting the day in the negative, you have the rest of the day to make up for it by targeting highly anti-inflammatory foods, such as fish — a small can of drained tuna in water has an IF rating of 698, so creating a small salad with spinach and tuna and a few other toppings like shredded carrots or a handful of nuts can quickly reverse the way your IF day is going.

The best way to know whether you're reaching your target — or even getting close — is to keep a food journal in which you write down the foods you eat and add up their ratings. There's no reason to keep the food journal indefinitely or even more than a few days — just use it to get in the habit of knowing what you're grabbing and ensuring that those foods are the right ones.

If you want to keep information at your fingertips, you can get an Inflammation Tracker application for the iPhone. Look for it at `www.lookingglass.mobi/if/`.

Looking up the numbers

Reinagel offers a small sample IF ratings list on her site, but for a more extensive list, check the website `http://nutritiondata.self.com`. It provides an area that allows you to enter a specific food and gives that food's nutritional breakdown, including the glycemic index and the inflammation factor rating. Table A-1 shows some common foods and their IF ratings.

Table A-1   Inflammation Factors of Common Foods

Food	Serving Size	Inflammation Factor (IF) Rating
French fries, fast food	Medium	−181
Bagel, plain	1 bagel	−180
Milk, lowfat (1%)	1 cup	−60
Butter	1 tablespoon	−48
Apple	1 medium	−30
Pork tenderloin, broiled or grilled	3 ounces	13
Broccoli, boiled	½ cup	60
Cantaloupe	1 cup	75
Carrot	1 raw	99
Salmon, Atlantic	3 ounces	493

Appendix B

Metric Conversion Guide

· ·

*N*ote: The recipes in this book weren't developed or tested using metric measurements. There may be some variation in quality when converting to metric units.

Common Abbreviations

Abbreviation(s)	What It Stands For
cm	Centimeter
C., c.	Cup
G, g	Gram
kg	Kilogram
L, l	Liter
lb.	Pound
mL, ml	Milliliter
oz.	Ounce
pt.	Pint
t., tsp.	Teaspoon
T., Tb., Tbsp.	Tablespoon

Volume

U.S. Units	Canadian Metric	Australian Metric
¼ teaspoon	1 milliliter	1 milliliter
½ teaspoon	2 milliliters	2 milliliters
1 teaspoon	5 milliliters	5 milliliters
1 tablespoon	15 milliliters	20 milliliters
¼ cup	50 milliliters	60 milliliters
⅓ cup	75 milliliters	80 milliliters
½ cup	125 milliliters	125 milliliters
⅔ cup	150 milliliters	170 milliliters
¾ cup	175 milliliters	190 milliliters
1 cup	250 milliliters	250 milliliters
1 quart	1 liter	1 liter
1½ quarts	1.5 liters	1.5 liters
2 quarts	2 liters	2 liters
2½ quarts	2.5 liters	2.5 liters
3 quarts	3 liters	3 liters
4 quarts (1 gallon)	4 liters	4 liters

Weight

U.S. Units	Canadian Metric	Australian Metric
1 ounce	30 grams	30 grams
2 ounces	55 grams	60 grams
3 ounces	85 grams	90 grams
4 ounces (¼ pound)	115 grams	125 grams
8 ounces (½ pound)	225 grams	225 grams
16 ounces (1 pound)	455 grams	500 grams (½ kilogram)

Length

Inches	Centimeters
0.5	1.5
1	2.5
2	5.0
3	7.5
4	10.0
5	12.5
6	15.0
7	17.5
8	20.5
9	23.0
10	25.5
11	28.0
12	30.5

Temperature (Degrees)

Fahrenheit	Celsius
32	0
212	100
250	120
275	140
300	150
325	160
350	180
375	190
400	200
425	220
450	230
475	240
500	260

Index

• E •

• F •

• O •

Apple & Macs

iPad For Dummies
978-0-470-58027-1

iPhone For Dummies,
4th Edition
978-0-470-87870-5

MacBook For Dummies, 3rd
Edition
978-0-470-76918-8

Mac OS X Snow Leopard For
Dummies
978-0-470-43543-4

Business

Bookkeeping For Dummies
978-0-7645-9848-7

Job Interviews
For Dummies,
3rd Edition
978-0-470-17748-8

Resumes For Dummies,
5th Edition
978-0-470-08037-5

Starting an
Online Business
For Dummies,
6th Edition
978-0-470-60210-2

Stock Investing
For Dummies,
3rd Edition
978-0-470-40114-9

Successful
Time Management
For Dummies
978-0-470-29034-7

Computer Hardware

BlackBerry
For Dummies,
4th Edition
978-0-470-60700-8

Computers For Seniors
For Dummies,
2nd Edition
978-0-470-53483-0

PCs For Dummies,
Windows
7 Edition
978-0-470-46542-4

Laptops For Dummies,
4th Edition
978-0-470-57829-2

Cooking & Entertaining

Cooking Basics
For Dummies,
3rd Edition
978-0-7645-7206-7

Wine For Dummies,
4th Edition
978-0-470-04579-4

Diet & Nutrition

Dieting For Dummies,
2nd Edition
978-0-7645-4149-0

Nutrition For Dummies,
4th Edition
978-0-471-79868-2

Weight Training
For Dummies,
3rd Edition
978-0-471-76845-6

Digital Photography

Digital SLR Cameras &
Photography For Dummies,
3rd Edition
978-0-470-46606-3

Photoshop Elements 8
For Dummies
978-0-470-52967-6

Gardening

Gardening Basics
For Dummies
978-0-470-03749-2

Organic Gardening
For Dummies,
2nd Edition
978-0-470-43067-5

Green/Sustainable

Raising Chickens
For Dummies
978-0-470-46544-8

Green Cleaning
For Dummies
978-0-470-39106-8

Health

Diabetes For Dummies,
3rd Edition
978-0-470-27086-8

Food Allergies
For Dummies
978-0-470-09584-3

Living Gluten-Free
For Dummies,
2nd Edition
978-0-470-58589-4

Hobbies/General

Chess For Dummies,
2nd Edition
978-0-7645-8404-6

Drawing
Cartoons & Comics
For Dummies
978-0-470-42683-8

Knitting For Dummies,
2nd Edition
978-0-470-28747-7

Organizing
For Dummies
978-0-7645-5300-4

Su Doku For Dummies
978-0-470-01892-7

Home Improvement

Home Maintenance
For Dummies,
2nd Edition
978-0-470-43063-7

Home Theater
For Dummies,
3rd Edition
978-0-470-41189-6

Living the
Country Lifestyle
All-in-One
For Dummies
978-0-470-43061-3

Solar Power Your Home
For Dummies,
2nd Edition
978-0-470-59678-4

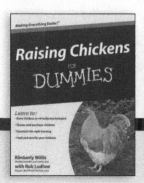
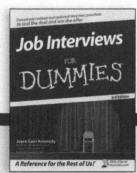
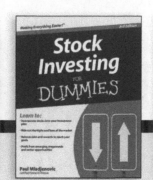
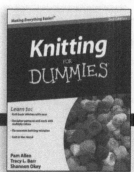

Available wherever books are sold. For more information or to order direct: U.S. customers visit www.dummies.com or call 1-877-762-2974.
U.K. customers visit www.wileyeurope.com or call (0) 1243 843291. Canadian customers visit www.wiley.ca or call 1-800-567-4797.

Internet

Blogging For Dummies,
3rd Edition
978-0-470-61996-4

eBay For Dummies,
6th Edition
978-0-470-49741-8

Facebook For Dummies,
3rd Edition
978-0-470-87804-0

Web Marketing
For Dummies,
2nd Edition
978-0-470-37181-7

WordPress
For Dummies,
3rd Edition
978-0-470-59274-8

Language & Foreign Language

French For Dummies
978-0-7645-5193-2

Italian Phrases
For Dummies
978-0-7645-7203-6

Spanish For Dummies,
2nd Edition
978-0-470-87855-2

Spanish
For Dummies,
Audio Set
978-0-470-09585-0

Math & Science

Algebra I
For Dummies,
2nd Edition
978-0-470-55964-2

Biology For Dummies,
2nd Edition
978-0-470-59875-7

Calculus For Dummies
978-0-7645-2498-1

Chemistry For Dummies
978-0-7645-5430-8

Microsoft Office

Excel 2010 For Dummies
978-0-470-48953-6

Office 2010 All-in-One
For Dummies
978-0-470-49748-7

Office 2010 For Dummies,
Book + DVD Bundle
978-0-470-62698-6

Word 2010 For Dummies
978-0-470-48772-3

Music

Guitar For Dummies,
2nd Edition
978-0-7645-9904-0

iPod & iTunes For
Dummies, 8th Edition
978-0-470-87871-2

Piano Exercises
For Dummies
978-0-470-38765-8

Parenting & Education

Parenting For Dummies,
2nd Edition
978-0-7645-5418-6

Type 1 Diabetes
For Dummies
978-0-470-17811-9

Pets

Cats For Dummies,
2nd Edition
978-0-7645-5275-5

Dog Training For Dummies,
3rd Edition
978-0-470-60029-0

Puppies For Dummies,
2nd Edition
978-0-470-03717-1

Religion & Inspiration

The Bible For Dummies
978-0-7645-5296-0

Catholicism For Dummies
978-0-7645-5391-2

Women in the Bible
For Dummies
978-0-7645-8475-6

Self-Help & Relationship

Anger Management
For Dummies
978-0-470-03715-7

Overcoming Anxiety
For Dummies,
2nd Edition
978-0-470-57441-6

Sports

Baseball
For Dummies,
3rd Edition
978-0-7645-7537-2

Basketball
For Dummies,
2nd Edition
978-0-7645-5248-9

Golf For Dummies,
3rd Edition
978-0-471-76871-5

Web Development

Web Design
All-in-One
For Dummies
978-0-470-41796-6

Web Sites
Do-It-Yourself
For Dummies,
2nd Edition
978-0-470-56520-9

Windows 7

Windows 7
For Dummies
978-0-470-49743-2

Windows 7
For Dummies,
Book + DVD Bundle
978-0-470-52398-8

Windows 7 All-in-One
For Dummies
978-0-470-48763-1

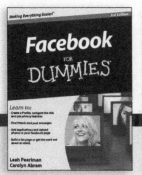

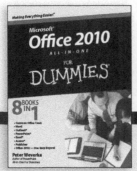

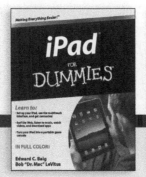

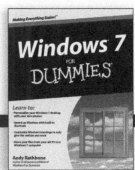

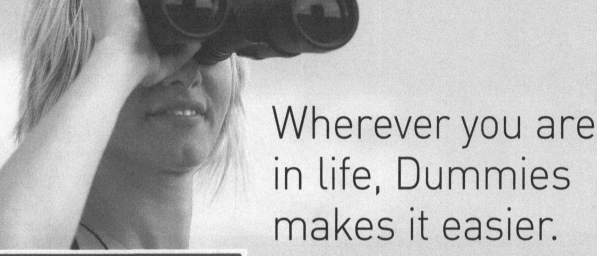
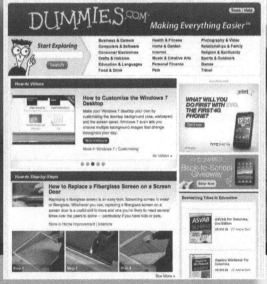
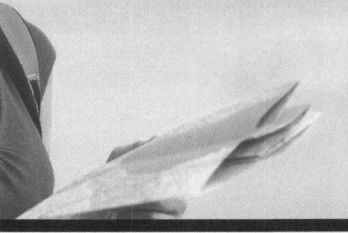

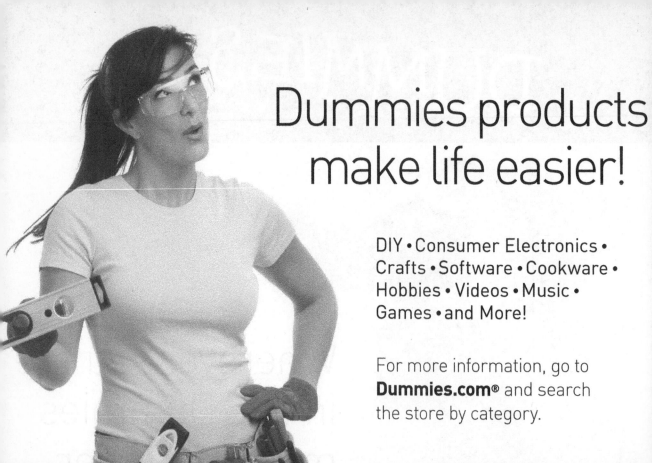
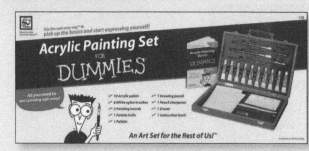
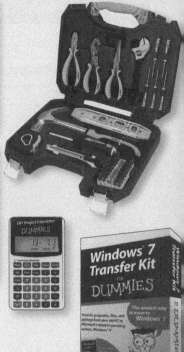
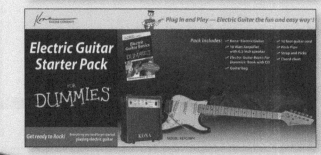
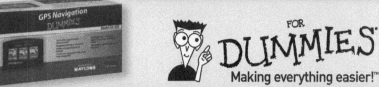